Nanotechnology Platforms for Antiviral Challenges

Nanotechnology provides an innovative platform for drug delivery and antiviral actions. This book discusses the utilization of nano-based formulations for the control of viral agents. The antiviral potential of green synthesized silver, chitosan nanoparticles encapsulating curcumin, photoinduced antiviral carbon nanohorns, and the role of carbon-based materials like fullerenes and carbon nanotubes in the repression of viral antigens are explained. The book also covers nanomaterial-based solutions for SARS-CoV-2 and other viral infections.

Features:

- Explains theory and practical applications of nanomaterials as antiviral agents.
- Reviews upscaling of nanomaterials from laboratory to fabrication stage.
- Illustrates nanocurcumin, silver nanoparticles, and carbon nanoparticles for biomedical applications.
- Highlights role of nanotechnology in effectively combating viral infections and pandemics.
- Includes case studies of specific pharma companies.

This book is aimed at researchers, graduate students in materials science, microbiology and virology, and pharmaceutical sciences.

Emerging Materials and Technologies

Series Editor: Boris I. Kharissov

The *Emerging Materials and Technologies* series is devoted to highlighting publications centered on emerging advanced materials and novel technologies. Attention is paid to those newly discovered or applied materials with potential to solve pressing societal problems and improve quality of life, corresponding to environmental protection, medicine, communications, energy, transportation, advanced manufacturing, and related areas.

The series takes into account that, under present strong demands for energy, material, and cost savings, as well as heavy contamination problems and worldwide pandemic conditions, the area of emerging materials and related scalable technologies is a highly interdisciplinary field, with the need for researchers, professionals, and academics across the spectrum of engineering and technological disciplines. The main objective of this book series is to attract more attention to these materials and technologies and invite conversation among the international R&D community.

Polymeric Biomaterials
Fabrication, Properties and Applications
Edited by Pooja Agarwal, Divya Bajpai Tripathy, Anjali Gupta and Bijoy Kumar Kuanr

Innovations in Green Nanoscience and Nanotechnology
Synthesis, Characterization, and Applications
Edited by Shrikaant Kulkarni

Sustainable Nanomaterials for the Construction Industry
Ghasan Fahim Huseien and Kwok Wei Shah

4D Imaging to 4D Printing
Biomedical Applications
Edited by Rupinder Singh

Emerging Nanomaterials for Catalysis and Sensor Applications
Edited by Anitha Varghese and Gurumurthy Hegde

Advanced Materials for a Sustainable Environment
Development Strategies and Applications
Edited by Naveen Kumar and Peter Ramashadi Makgwane

Nanomaterials from Renewable Resources for Emerging Applications
Edited by Sandeep S. Ahankari, Amar K. Mohanty, and Manjusri Misra

Multifunctional Polymeric Foams
Advancements and Innovative Approaches
Edited by Soney C George and Resmi B. P.

Nanotechnology Platforms for Antiviral Challenges
Fundamentals, Applications and Advances
Edited by Soney C George and Ann Rose Abraham

Carbon-Based Conductive Polymer Composites
Processing, Properties, and Applications in Flexible Strain Sensors
Dong Xiang

Nanocarbons
Preparation, Assessments, and Applications
Ashwini P. Alegaonkar and Prashant S. Alegaonkar

Emerging Applications of Carbon Nanotubes and Graphene
Edited by Bhanu Pratap Singh and Kiran M. Subhedar
For more information about this series, please visit:
www.routledge.com/Emerging-Materials-and-Technologies/book-series/CRCEMT

Nanotechnology Platforms
for Antiviral Challenges

Fundamentals, Applications and Advances

Edited by

Soney C George

and

Ann Rose Abraham

CRC Press
Taylor & Francis Group
Boca Raton London New York

CRC Press is an imprint of the
Taylor & Francis Group, an **informa** business

First edition published 2023
by CRC Press
6000 Broken Sound Parkway NW, Suite 300, Boca Raton, FL 33487-2742

and by CRC Press
4 Park Square, Milton Park, Abingdon, Oxon, OX14 4RN

CRC Press is an imprint of Taylor & Francis Group, LLC

ISBN: 9781032152301 (hbk)
ISBN: 9781032152325 (pbk)
ISBN: 9781003243175 (ebk)

DOI: 10.1201/9781003243175

Typeset in Times
by Deanta Global Publishing Services, Chennai, India

Contents

Editor Biographies

Soney C George, PhD, is Dean of Research and Director of the Amal Jyothi Centre for Nanoscience and Technology, Kerala, India. He is a Fellow of the Royal Society of Chemistry, London, UK, and a recipient of the "Best Researcher of the Year" award in 2018 from APJ Abdul Kalam Technological University, Thiruvananthapuram, India. He has also received awards such as National Technical Teacher's Award 2022 of AICTE and the best faculty award from the Indian Society for Technical Education, best citation award from the *International Journal of Hydrogen Energy*, a fast-track award of young scientists by the Department of Science and Technology, India, and an Indian young scientist award instituted by the Indian Science Congress Association. He did his postdoctoral studies at the University of Blaise Pascal, France, and Inha University, South Korea. He has published and presented almost 200 publications in journals and at conferences. His major research fields are polymer nanocomposites, polymer membranes, polymer tribology, pervaporation, and supercapacitors. He has guided eight PhD scholars and 112 student projects.

Ann Rose Abraham, PhD, received her MSc, M. Phil and PhD degrees in Physics from School of Pure and Applied Physics, Mahatma Gandhi University, Kerala, India. She has expertise in the field of materials science, nanomagnetic materials, multiferroics, and polymeric nanocomposites, etc. She has research experience at various national institutes like the Bose Institute, SAHA Institute of Nuclear Physics, UGC-DAE CSR Centre, Kolkata and collaborations with various international laboratories like University of Johannesburg, South Africa, Institute of Physics Belgrade, etc. She is the recipient of a Young Researcher award in Physics, a prestigious forum to showcase intellectual capability. Dr. Ann is currently working as an Assistant Professor, S.H. College, Thevara, India. She is a frequent speaker at national and international conferences. She has four years of teaching experience at various levels. She has authored many book chapters and edited books with Taylor and Francis, Elsevier, etc. She has a good number of publications to her credit in many peer reviewed high impact journals of international repute.

Contributors

Ann Rose Abraham
Department of Physics, Sacred Heart College, Thevara, India

Sartaj Ahmad
Department of Physics, AAAM, Government Degree College Bemina, Cluster University Srinagar, India

Mohammad Ashfaq
Advanced Ceramics and Nanotechnology Laboratory, Department of Materials Engineering, Faculty of Engineering, University of Concepción, Chile; School of Life Science, BS Abdur Rahman Crescent Institute of Science and Technology, Chennai, India

Amala Rose Augustine
Department of Physics, Sacred Heart College, Thevara, India

Tabassum Khair Barbhuiya
Department of Pharmaceutical Sciences, Drug Discovery Research Laboratory, Assam University, Silchar, India

Yogesh Bharat Dalvi
Pushpagiri Research Centre, Pushpagiri, Institute of Medical Science & Research, Tiruvalla, Kerala, India

Nirupam Das
Department of Pharmaceutical Sciences, Drug Discovery Research Laboratory, Assam University, Silchar, India

Tannu Garg
Amity Institute of Applied Sciences, Amity University Uttar Pradesh, Noida, India

Soney C George
Dean of Research and Director, Amal Jyothi Centre for Nanoscience and Technology, Kerala, India

Tejendra Gupta
Amity Institute of Applied Sciences, Amity University Uttar Pradesh, Noida, India

Md. Amzad Hossain
Department of Physics, AAAM, Government Degree College Bemina, Cluster University Srinagar, India

Sara Jones
Pathogen Biology Group, Rajiv Gandhi Centre for Biotechnology (National Institute under the Department of Biotechnology, Govt. of India), Thiruvananthapuram, Kerala, India

Binu Prakash
Institute of Physiology, Czech Academy of Sciences, Czech Republic

Partha Palit
Department of Pharmaceutical Sciences, Drug Discovery Research Laboratory, Assam University, Silchar, India

Gad Elsayed Mohamed Salem
Reef Biology Research Group,
    Department of Marine Science,
    Faculty of Science, Chulalongkorn
    University, Bangkok, Thailand

and

Department of Microbiology, Egyptian
    Drug Authority (EDA), Formerly
    National Organization for Drug
    Control and Research (NODCAR),
    Giza, Egypt

Akhila Velappan Savithri
Pathogen Biology Group, Rajiv Gandhi
    Centre for Biotechnology (National
    Institute under the Department of
    Biotechnology, Govt. of India),
    Thiruvananthapuram, Kerala, India

Gaurav Sharma
Amity Institute of Applied Sciences,
    Amity University Uttar Pradesh,
    Noida, India

Mir, Vipin Shrotriya
Department of Physics, AAAM,
    Government Degree College Bemina,
    Cluster University Srinagar, India

Karthika Suryaletha
Pathogen Biology Group, Rajiv Gandhi
    Centre for Biotechnology (National
    Institute under the Department of
    Biotechnology, Govt. of India),
    Thiruvananthapuram, Kerala, India

Neetu Talreja
Advanced Ceramics and
    Nanotechnology Laboratory,
    Department of Materials
    Engineering, Faculty of Engineering,
    University of Concepción, Chile

Ruby Varghese
Department of Chemistry, School
    of Sciences, Jain Deemed to be
    University, Bangalore, Karnataka,
    India

Sasidharan Venkataramanan
Department of Biotechnology, School
    of Chemical and Biotechnology,
    SASTRA DEEMED University,
    Thanjavur, Tamilnadu, India

Rohit Verma
Amity Institute of Applied Sciences,
    Amity University Uttar Pradesh,
    Noida, India

Namitha Vijay
Pushpagiri Research Centre,
    Pushpagiri Institute of Medical
    Science & Research, Tiruvalla,
    Kerala, India

Mangalaraja Ramalinga Viswanathan
Advanced Ceramics and
    Nanotechnology Laboratory,
    Department of Materials
    Engineering, Faculty of Engineering,
    University of Concepción, Chile;
    Technological Development Unit
    (UDT), University of Concepcion,
    Coronel Industrial Park, Coronel,
    Chile

M Burhanuz Zaman
Department of Physics, AAAM
    Government Degree College Bemina,
    Cluster University Srinagar, India

Preface

Nanotechnology offers viable methods to address frequent viral infections in human beings. Antiviral therapeutics has emerged as a successful warrior against the challenges posed by viruses inside the body. The solubility and toxicity of antiviral drugs are of serious concern during administering drugs while nanotechnology has revolutionized the properties of drugs so that their effectiveness and selectivity toward viral cells has tremendously improved. The advent of the COVID-19 pandemic has accelerated the development of antiviral materials such as drugs, personal protective devices, etc based on nanoparticles, nanomaterials, polymer-based nanocomposites, etc.

In this book the current status of effective utilization of principles of nanotechnology in antiviral applications is narrated.

Chapter 1 gives an insight into the antiviral potential of functional nanoparticles. Chapter 2 provides an overview of the applications of nanotechnology in the antimicrobial field. Chapter 3 summarizes the role of antiviral polymers in food safety related applications while Chapter 4 specifically focused on antiviral biopolymers in food packaging applications. Toxicology of nanoparticle-based pharmaceuticals is discussed in Chapter 5. Chapter 6 examines the role of quantum dots as antiviral agents. Chapter 7 narrates the effectiveness of nanoparticles as antiviral agents in combating pandemics and Chapter 8 discusses the role of nanotechnology in antiviral treatment against the current coronavirus (SARS-CoV-2).

This book covers recent advances in the field of antiviral applications. It serves as an invaluable guide to professionals, researchers, industrialists, graduate students, and senior undergraduates in the fields of virology, antiviral materials, materials science, nano devices, polymer chemistry, nanoscience, and those who work in similar areas or are interested in the field of antiviral materials.

All chapters were contributed by renowned professionals from academic, industry, and government laboratories from various countries and were peer reviewed in accordance with the guidelines utilized elsewhere by top-rated journals. The editors would like to thank all contributors for believing in this endeavour, sharing their views and precious time, and obtaining documents. The editors would like to express their gratitude to the external reviewers whose contributions helped to improve the quality of this book and the publishing team for their constant encouragement and support.

Editors

Dr. Soney C George and Dr. Ann Rose Abraham

1 A Reflection of Antiviral Potential of Functional Nanoparticles

Amala Rose Augustine, Ann Rose Abraham,
and Soney C George

CONTENTS

1.1 INTRODUCTION

The equilibrium of life of the entire human race was ruined by the outbreak of the COVID-19 pandemic caused by the novel coronavirus in the year 2019. The infections caused by these pathogens are affecting the world's health and economy. Viral pandemics like H1N1, H2N2 (1956–1958), H3N3 (1968), flu, Ebola (1975 to present), SARS (2009), MERS (2012 till now) are nightmares created by these pathogens (Reina et al., 2020). They are among the leading causes of disability, death, and social and economic problems (Morens et al., 2004). They are parasites with RNA or DNA and a protein coat (Milovanovic et al., 2017). Even with the available vaccines and

DOI: 10.1201/9781003243175-1

1

antibiotics, we were unable to prevent the surge in infections. There are numerous similar viral agents causing disastrous diseases leading to increased mortality rates. The available techniques are inadequate for fighting the pathogens and research is being undertaken on a worldwide scale for the development of new antiviral strategies. Such research also aims to determine preventive measures in order to reduce harm due to viral diseases. There are technologies that slow down the spread of infection. But their high cost limits the usage of these facilities. Thus, we have an obvious urgency to develop new strategies to fight these pathogens (Reina et al., 2020).

The interaction of these pathogens with the host cells occurs in multiple steps. Initially it binds to the host cell and then enters the cytoplasm by several mechanisms. This is followed by the liberation of the viral genome from the protective capsid and after a series of events the replication of the genome takes place followed by the release of the newly generated virions. Each step of the replication process can be targeted for producing effective antiviral agents (Galdiero et al., 2011). The high rate of mutations exhibited by these creatures makes the development of vaccines difficult. They exhibit notable potential to adapt to the host, to parasitize a newly found host, and to overcome the antiviral measures taken through genetic adaptability (Domingo, 2010). Lack of proper vaccines to prevent these infections urges the development of efficient drugs to avert the entry and replication of these killers into the cells. A few chemical drugs capable of this like acyclovir, ganciclovir etc. were developed and research has revealed their numerous side effects (Nitsche et al., 2014). Low solubility and retentivity of these drugs are also drawbacks associated with their use. The pathogens developing antibiotic resistance, the abuse of these drugs, and various environmental hazards resulting from their usage are also factors limiting their usage. The development of broad-spectrum antiviral agents is also difficult as the replication process differs from one virus to another.

Antiviral agents can be broadly classified into two, namely virostatic and virucidal (Cagno et al., 2018). Virostatic substances act on early stages of infection, mainly by preventing viral binding and entry to the cells while virucidal materials cause the deactivation of viruses permanently (Sengupta and Hussain, 2020). The emerging nanoscience came up with a solution for this issue by reporting the extraordinary ability exhibited by some nanoparticles to fight these pathogens (Russo et al., 2014, Hang et al., 2015). The antimicrobial activity of these particles towards a wide spectrum of pathogens including fungi, viruses, and bacteria has been inspected. Nanoparticles with a size in the order of nanometres interact very well through biochemical interaction with nanosized viruses (Sengupta and Hussain, 2020). A small size, large surface area-to-volume ratio (Ingle et al., 2014), and a surface that can be modified according to the requirements etc. are just a few among the unique characteristics that make nanoparticles the best choice for developing antiviral agents. These particles can be modified to incorporate multiple antiviral agents. Various carbon nanoparticles like fullerene, carbon nanotubes, graphene oxide, metal nanoparticles like gold, silver, zinc, different polymer nanoparticles etc. are extensively researched and employed in antiviral applications.

The contributions from the world of little particles to fight the little creatures include probes like biosensors using nanotechnology for pathogen detection (Caygill et al., 2010, Cao et al., 2011, Chen et al., 2012, Daaboul et al., 2010), inhibitors acting as barriers for production of multiple copies of virus in infected cells (White et al., 2018), some fluorescent nanoprobes for detecting infected cells (Pan et al., 2014, Zhang et al., 2013b), drug carrier-delivery mechanisms for certain antiviral agents (Falanga et al., 2011, Hallaj et al., 2010) etc. Their ability to act on specific targets helps in protecting uninfected cells (Milovanovic et al., 2017).

Nanotheranostics can be described as one of the most dynamic fields in treating various pathological conditions. Research is currently taking place with the aim of completing both diagnostic as well as therapeutic processes in one, multifunctional nano-platform. Recently theranostic particles were employed in drug and vaccine delivery and in tracking infections and treatments (Fouad, 2021). The physiochemical features including size, charge, easy techniques involved in the synthesis and the ability of targeted drug delivery make multifunctional nanoparticles suitable candidates for developing theranostic agents (Singh et al., 2017a). While designing a theranostic-based nano-platform, the three elements that need to be considered include the nanocarrier, therapeutic agent, and imaging agent (Madamsetty et al., 2019). Theranostic activities were exhibited by biosynthesized nanoparticles carrying therapeutic molecules with imaging agents (Ma et al., 2012). Hence there is a scope for developing nanoparticles with the ability to diagnose and treat viral infections. The most common theranostic agents used today are gold (Liu, 2018) and magnetic nanoparticles (Singh and Sahoo, 2014). Magnetic nanoparticles are largely used as contrast media in MRI or as drug carriers.

In this chapter the characteristics of various nanoparticles including metallic nanoparticles, carbon nanoparticles, polymeric nanoparticles, and various other functional nanoparticles are explored for their antiviral potential. The mechanisms of viral inhibition by nanoparticles are summarized. We aim to spur the interest of researchers to make advanced discoveries in the field of antiviral potential of nanoparticles through this chapter.

1.2 FUNCTIONAL NANOPARTICLES AND THEIR ANTIVIRAL CAPACITY

Nanomaterials exhibit great functionality and therapeutic potential as antiviral agents, inhibiting the activity of viruses. In this chapter, we briefly describe the most common types of nanomaterials that are used for antiviral applications. The virucidal properties of carbon nanoparticles, metal nanoparticles, polymeric nanoparticles, and other functional nanoparticles are summarized. The different classes of functional nanoparticles exhibiting antiviral potential are demonstrated in Figure 1.1.

1.2.1 Carbon Nanoparticles

1.2.1.1 Carbon Quantum Dots

Quantum dots (QDs) can be defined as semiconductor crystals, exhibiting size dependent electrical and optical properties (Michalet et al., 2005). Due to their

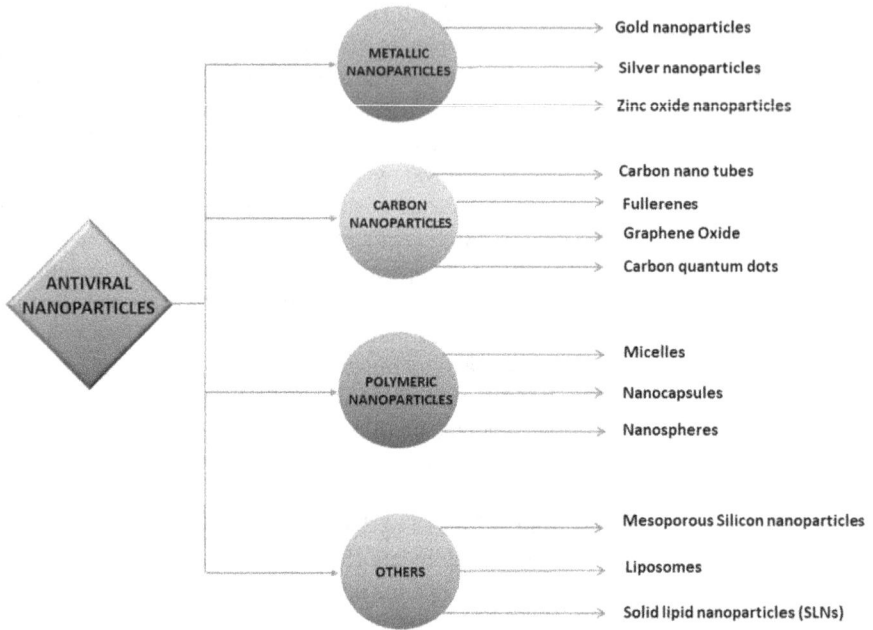

FIGURE 1.1   Schematic of nanoparticles with antiviral potential

luminescent properties, they are predominately employed in cell labelling, virus detection etc. (Chen et al., 2018, Wu et al., 2016). QDs exhibit fluorescent properties and are used for bioimaging purposes and their solubility is enhanced in aqueous buffers (Malik et al., 2013).

The efficiency of glutathione (GSH)-capped CdTe QDs on the pseudorabies virus (PRV) was investigated by Du et al. and it was found that the virus was prevented from entering the host cell due to QDs. They also identified how the antiviral activity of these particles varied with variation in size and charge i.e., positively charged larger QDs are the best (Du et al., 2015). Antiretroviral drug saquinavir and transferrin – a biorecognition molecule – were conjugated with QDs for enhancing drug delivery into the brain for treating cells infected by HIV-1. It was reported that the drug concentration that reached the target was high. This was due to the ability of drug-doped quantum dots to move across the blood brain barrier and the result implies that it can be employed in treating neural AIDS and other issues (Yong et al., 2012).

Small carbon nanoparticles of a particle size under 10 nm are called carbon nanodots or carbon quantum dots. These lower toxic carbon dots (CDs) were examined for their action on viral reproduction with DNA and RNA virus as test models and the results indicated the prevention of reproduction by QDs (Chen and Liang, 2020). The increased production of interferons (IFNs) that defended the virus upon the application of CDs due to the expression of interference stimulating genes (ISGs) was also reported (Liu et al., 2017). The infectivity of various non-enveloped viruses was found to be suppressed by benzoxazine monomer-derived carbon dots (BZM-CDs) developed by Huang et al. by inhibiting their interaction with the host cell. These particles directly bind to the virions and prevent the initial phase of interaction between the virus and host cell (Huang et al., 2019).

Surface-modified CDs exhibit better antiviral actions. CDs functionalized with boronic acid or amine-inhibiting herpes simplex virus type 1 (HSV-1) is an example. Studies reveal that the initial stages of the viral entry into the cell get obstructed (Barras et al., 2016). Ethylenediamine/citric acid on hydrothermal carbonization yields carbon dots which inhibit the coronavirus. CQDs derived from 4-amino-phenylboronic acid exhibited the inactivation of human coronavirus concentration dependently, by interacting with the receptors and replication process (Łoczechin et al., 2019).

Curcumin has been proved to be effective in combatting viruses. Considering the application of Chinese medicines in fighting the virus, the curcumin-modified cationic carbon dots (CCM-CDs) synthesized by Du et al. exhibited the efficient inhibition of the proliferation of the porcine epidemic diarrhoea virus (PEDV) when compared to non-modified CDs (Ting et al., 2018). The production of interferon-stimulating genes (ISGs) and proinflammatory cytokines were stimulated and triggered by the application of these CCM-CDs leading to the suppression of viral replication. The QDs developed with glycyrrhizic acid (a Chinese medicine), which are highly biocompatible, possessed broad antiviral capacity with high efficiency to prevent various stages of infection like invasion, replication, reducing infection etc. (Tong et al., 2020). These examples show that CDs and Chinese medicines together can create great advancements in the fight against viruses.

1.2.1.2 Graphene Oxide

Graphene is identified to be a good candidate for destroying viruses. Its efficiency to destroy different types of viruses is well observed. Song et al. discuss the ability of graphene oxide (GO) in the detection and disinfection of viruses (Song et al., 2015). The efficiency of disinfection is highly temperature dependent. The evident viricidal effect can be easily extended to a broad spectrum of applications in the antiviral field. Also, their amphiphilic nature allows the attachment of hydrophobic and hydrophilic substances (Neto and Fileti, 2018). GO has been reported to exhibit significant antiviral activity. The ability of GO to suppress the activity of the pseudorabies virus (PRV) and intestinal infection causing porcine epidemic diarrhoea virus (PEDV) was examined and was attributed to being caused by the single layer composition and the negative charge (Ye et al., 2015).

Pokhrel et al. recommended the development of disinfectants based on graphene to prevent the Ebola epidemic after examining the interactions between graphene and viral proteins (Pokhrel et al., 2018, Chakravarty and Vora, 2021). Deokar et al. used reduced graphene oxide to functionalize sulphonated magnetic nanoparticles. These nanoparticles (SMRGO) were found capable of entrapping and destroying a large number of viruses (Deokar et al., 2017). Curcumin being an antiviral agent, curcumin-loaded graphene oxide was highly effective in inhibiting the respiratory syncytial virus (RSV). Inactivation of the virus, hindering its attachment to the host cell, preventing its replication etc. are some of the methodologies exhibited by the functionalized graphene oxide to fight viral infections (Yang et al., 2017). Further studies conducted proved the effectiveness of these particles against viral infections, mainly by blocking them from getting attached to host cells. These particles can be used for developing safer drugs which are more efficient with least adverse effects.

Composite formed from GO and sulphonated partially reduced GO mimicked the cell surface receptor heparan sulphate, prevented herpes simplex virus type-1 (HSV-1), and exhibited no cytotoxic effect (Sametband et al., 2014). GO and Ag NPs can be combined to form composites which exhibit enhanced antiviral activity when compared to their individual activities (Chen et al., 2016). Novel duck reovirus (NDRV) disease, affecting poultry, is found to be reduced upon the application of hypericin (HY)-loaded GO, due to viral inactivation and the prevention of viral attachment (Du et al., 2019). Drug development from graphene oxide Quantum Dots (GQDs) is under research. The development of anti-HIV agents using GQDs conjugated with inhibitors by Iannazzo is an example (Iannazzo et al., 2018). Fluorine-functionalized QDs are also used to prevent the aggregation of human islet amyloid polypeptide (hIAPP) (Yousaf et al., 2017). Thus, graphene quantum dot-based inhibitors are employed against protein aggregation which can lead to serious diseases.

1.2.1.3 Carbon Nanotubes

Carbon nanotubes (CNTs) are hollow cylindrical nanomaterials developed from graphene sheets. Their applications in biomedical fields are restricted due to high pulmonary toxicity and hydrophobicity (Shao et al., 2013). Pulmonary toxicity resulting from usage of SWCNT and an increase in influenza A infection was explained by Chen et al. (Chen et al., 2017). But functionalization can notably reduce this toxicity.

Multi-walled nanotubes (MWNTs) conjugated with Protoporphyrin IX (PPIX) was recognized as an excellent agent resulting in the inactivation of a wide range of viruses (Kumar et al., 2014). Oxidised CNTs displayed inhibitory activity towards the HIV virus (Iannazzo et al., 2015). Grover et al. put forward the usage of MWCNTs for immobilizing AcT (perhydrolase) and incorporating this into paints that are latex-based and used in forming catalytic coatings, which exhibited a reduction of the influenza virus (Grover et al., 2013). MWCNT-DENV3 developed by functionalization of MWCNT with a recombinant dengue envelope was observed to be an efficient candidate for a dengue vaccine (Versiani et al., 2017).

Functionalized CNTs are also employed to deliver drugs. The unique architecture and properties of CNTs make them suitable candidates for this purpose (Ezzati et al., 2011). Andrade et al. in the review on nanostructured vaccines, discuss the engagement of CNTs for transporting peptides for vaccination (Andrade et al., 2017). HSV-1, when treated with acyclovir delivered by oxidised CNTs functionalized with cyclodextrin, a much higher anti replicative effect was observed when compared to other drugs (Iannazzo et al., 2014). The conjugation of antimicrobial peptides (AMPs) with CNT at a very low concentration led to the easy activation of AMPs (Pradhan et al., 2017). The antagonistic interaction of CNTs to the target proteins of HIV was reported by Navanietha et al. (Navanietha et al., 2014). SWCNTs decorated with metal and combined to hydrogen peroxide were found to be effective in fighting viruses. Studies showcased SWCNT as a substrate with high potential to confine, inactivate, and manage viruses. These metal-decorated SWCNTs can be used to develop self-cleaning respirators and devices to detect viruses (Aasi et al., 2020).

A nanofilter to remove virus from water was developed using CNT and was tested for its efficiency on the MS2 virus (Mostafavi et al., 2009). Yeh et al. introduced a CNT-based portable microfluid platform for the capture of viruses by the rapid enrichment and optical identification of viruses. The SERS platform exhibited high efficiency in identifying a broad spectrum of viruses (Yeh et al., 2020). Plasmonic nanoparticle- (gold) decorated CNTs were used for developing a plasmon-assisted fluoro-immunoassay (PAFI), which was found to be excellent in detecting the influenza virus (Lee et al., 2015). Tam et al. developed a DNA sensor for detecting a label-free influenza virus (Tam et al., 2009). MWCNT complex with CAR protein – a human cellular receptor – was found to be highly efficient in detecting environmental adenoviruses, hence it can be used to construct biosensors (Zhang et al., 2007).

1.2.1.4 Fullerenes

Fullerenes are nanosized hollow spheres made up of 60 carbon atoms. The size, hydrophobicity, and unique structure of fullerenes make them the best candidate for therapeutic applications. They are the most attractive carbon nanomaterials for antiviral potential. The low solubility exhibited by pure fullerene led to research on functionalization (Reina et al., 2020).

Fullerenes, due to their hydrophobicity, have the ability to inhibit the HIV virus by binding with the HIV proteases, particularly its hydrophobic cavity, which leads to the inhibition of virus multiplication (Bondavalli et al., 2018). Their biological features like unique architecture and antioxidant capacity are responsible for antiviral activity. The studies suggested that the antiviral activity is dependent on the substituent position of fullerenes and positive charges in close proximity to the fullerenes' cage. Derivatives of transfullerenes were found to be more dynamic than the cis, while equatorial ones were totally inactive. HIV 1 and HIV 2 were found to be inhibited by fulleropyrrolidines containing two ammonium groups (Bakry et al., 2007). The human cytomegalovirus and HIV were found to be inhibited by amino acid derivatives of fullerene C60 (ADF) (Kotelnikova et al., 2003). The pharmaceutical importance of fullerenes and their derivatives' are great due to the fact that they are poorly immunogenetic. Enveloped viruses are inhibited by water soluble C 60 derivatives (Bakry et al., 2007).

Attempts were made to prepare a wide spectrum antiviral agent against enveloped viruses like Ebola, Zika etc. Different glycofullerenes were prepared by combining different numbers of mannose with fullerene and were tested for activity against Ebola infection. The inhibiting capacities was observed to vary among different species prepared. More studies were conducted on these glycofullerenes and their ability to act as an antiviral agent against a large spectrum of viruses was made obvious. The low toxicity of glycofullerenes was also proved. (Reina et al., 2020, Nierengarten and Nierengarten, 2014). Glycofullerenes do not possess any virucidal effect. Their potential to inhibit viral activity lies in their ability to prevent viral entry into the cells. Hence, sufficient concentration of these glycofullerenes is required in order to ensure their shielding capacity (Reina et al., 2020).

1.2.2 METAL NANOPARTICLES

1.2.2.1 Silver Nanoparticles

Being well known for a wide variety of properties like antifungal, anti-cancer, antibacterial etc., silver nanoparticles (Ag NPs) are used extensively (Lü et al., 2017, Kuppusamy et al., 2015). But their antiviral effects are still under research. The ability of these particles to interfere in a few stages of viral replication was noticed (Milovanovic et al., 2017). Galdiero et al. have reviewed Ag NPs potential as antiviral agents (Galdiero et al., 2011). The antiviral action of Ag NPs was ascribed due to the inhibition of viral entry i.e., it acts as a viral entry inhibitor (Lara et al., 2010a). Studies on the Peste des petits ruminants virus (PPRV) inhibition (Khandelwal et al., 2014) and vaccinia inhibition (Trefry and Wooley, 2013) by Ag NPs revealed that Ag NPs viral inhibition is by preventing viral entry to host cells and that they lack virus-killing effects. Alternately, these NPs can be combined with the viral nucleic acid and can make it inactive or prevent its replication (Reina et al., 2020, Lu et al., 2008, Chen et al., 2013).

The quasi-spherical silver nanoparticles prepared from the roots of a plant exhibited antiviral properties against the influenza A virus (Sreekanth et al., 2018). Haggag et al. reported the ability of Ag NPs synthesized through green synthesis methods from lamapranthuscoccineus and Malephora lutea to inhibit the hepatitis A virus (HAV-10), herpes simplex virus (HSV-1), and CoxB4 viruses (Haggag et al., 2019). Elechiguerra et al. studied how Ag NPs interact with HIV 1 and found that the interaction is size dependent (Elechiguerra et al., 2005). The inhibition of HIV-1 with silver nanoparticles works by hindering the entry of the virus and by interrupting gp120-CD4 interaction; these particles are also capable of inhibiting the post-entry stages of the virus (Galdiero et al., 2011). Hepatitis B Virus (HBV) replication was observed to be prevented by AgNPs and the antiviral mechanism was hypothesized (Lu et al., 2008).

Silver nanoparticle-coated polyvinylpyrrolidone (PVP) is effective in inhibiting viral activity. Lara et al. found that PVP-coated silver nanoparticles, when formulated into replens gel, was effective in controlling the spread of HIV-1 and isolated cell-free HIV-1. This formulation exhibited a long-lasting protective effect (Lara et al., 2010b). The cytoprotective and anti-HIV 1 activity of Ag NPs synthesized from heps buffer was discovered by Sun et al. (Sun et al., 2005). A similar inhibition was observed with nanoparticles reduced with a citrate solution with NaBH4. Polyurethane condoms (PUCs) coated with Ag NPs were active against HIV 1 and HSV. The T-tropic and M-tropic strains of HIV-1 exhibited high sensitivity towards them (Fayaz et al., 2012). Respiratory syncytial virus (RSV) inhibition by Ag NPs capped by different proteins like bovine serum albumin (BSA), PVP, and RF412 (F-protein) were evaluated. BSA-conjugated Ag NPs interacted with the virus but without exhibiting any particular association, RF412-conjugated NPs floated freely without any attachment, while PVP-coated Ag NPs exhibited binding to viral surfaces. And these conjugates exhibited only low cytotoxicity. Thus Sun et al. demonstrated that capping with suitable substances can reduce the toxicity of certain nanoparticles by masking those which are otherwise toxic. Hence, PVP-coated Ag NPs are proven to be promising candidates for RSV treatment (Sun et al., 2008).

Suppression of monkey pox virus (MPV) infection by silver nanoparticles and polysaccharide-coated silver nanoparticles was discovered (Rogers et al., 2008). HSV 1 infection was found to be prevented by Ag NPs functionalized with mercaptoethane sulfonate (MES) as it inhibited viral entry to the cells. The nanoparticles inhibited viral entry by competing with viruses to bind with the cell surface heparan sulphate (HS) (Baram et al., 2009). Suppression of HIV influenza A virus activity by AgNp-chitosan composite was studied by Mori et al. and they found that the composite was antiviral and activity surged with a concentration of nanoparticles, while chitosan alone had no effect on viral activities. They also observed the variation of activity depended on the size of the nanoparticles, that stronger activity was exhibited by small particles (Mori et al., 2013).

The efficiency of curcumin-modified Ag NPs (c-Ag NPs) to suppress respiratory syncytial virus (RSV) infection was investigated by Yang et al. and they confirmed its viricidal ability (Yang et al., 2016). Tacaribe virus (TCRV), which is not a human pathogen from the family Arenaviridae, and exhibiting similarities to few human pathogens, was found to be reduced by Ag NPs and it was also noted that coating nanoparticles with polysaccharides reduced the toxicity but also interfered with the antiviral mechanism, reducing it (Speshock et al., 2010). Orlowski et al. found that silver nanoparticles sized 33 nm, modified with tannic acid – a polyphenol derived from plants – can act as an efficient antiviral microbicide which can be employed to develop resistance against HSV 2 on mucosal tissues (Orłowski et al., 2018). This inhibition was found to be caused by the direct blocking of viral entry to cells and inflammation suppression. Bio-nanocomposites of Ag NPs decorated with polyquaternary phosphonium oligochitosans exhibited synergistic antiviral potential towards the hepatitis A virus (HAV), coxsackievirus B4 (CoxB4), and norovirus (NoV) infections (Sofy et al., 2019).

Antiviral effects of the combination of two nanoparticles, graphene oxide together with silver nanoparticles on enveloped and non-enveloped viruses, were studied and the increased efficiency of the combination was observed (Chen et al., 2016). The enveloped feline coronavirus (F CoV) can be destroyed by rupturing it with GO Ag NPs. Sinclair et al. discuss the importance of various capping agents on Ag NPs, that capping agents decide the antiviral activity of the material. Six differently capped nanoparticles were tested for their ability on MS2 bacteriophages. The important role played by surface charge on virucidal activity was demonstrated, that the most negative nanoparticles repelled negative viruses without any kind of interaction, while the NPs with the highest positive charge exhibited highest reduction (Sinclair et al., 2021). Ag NPs are suitable candidates for water treatment to prevent waterborne viral infections.

The capability of nanoparticles to deliver antiviral peptide Flupep was analysed by Alghrair et al. and the enhanced antiviral ability of Flupep against the influenza virus was observed (Alghrair et al., 2019). The H1N1 influenza virus was found to be inhibited more efficiently by an anti-influenza drug loaded with Ag NPs and the virus was also inactivated (Lin et al., 2017).

A limitation in using these Ag NPs in viricidal actions is that it is formulated in a liquid state. One advance in overcoming this is that of hydrogel preparation. Tannic acid-modified Ag NPs hydrogel for the herpes simplex virus (HSV) infections is an example (Szymańska et al., 2018). This TA-Ag NPs gel was modified by encapsulating it in a 3-D crosslinked polymer matrix, improving its action. These hydrogels are not only good carriers, but also efficient wide spectrum antiviral agents (Dey et al., 2018).

Though silver nanoparticle is recognized as a candidate with great antiviral potential, the challenges like self-agglomeration and pollution issues limit its large-scale usage. But the modification of Ag NPs with substances like PVP and other masking materials can help to overcome these issues. But this can also contribute to the reduction of the antiviral potential.

1.2.2.2   Gold Nanoparticles

Gold nanoparticles (Au NPs) are biocompatible colloidal nanosized particles of gold. The surface plasmon resonance (SPR) exhibited by these nanoparticles contributes to their extensive scientific and technological application in diverse areas. These particles are used in cancer studies and as antibacterial as well as antiviral agents as they can easily detect DNA, virus, bacteria etc. The advancements in the field of cancer treatment by application of Au NPs are highly notable (Huang and El-Sayed, 2010). The quantum size effect exhibited by gold nanoparticles makes them good candidates for nanomedicine and other biomedical applications. They exhibit low toxicity when compared to silver. They are attributed to exhibit display effects on various pathogens. The herpes simplex virus (HSP) was reported to be inhibited and controlled using mono-dispersed quasi-spherical gold nanoparticles (Halder et al., 2018). The dimensions and morphology of these particles are the key factors that make these particles antivirally active (Reina et al., 2020).

Porous Au NPs were found to be successful in preventing the influenza virus by cleaving the disulphide bond of Hemagglutinin (HA), a viral surface protein that helps in the fusion process (Kim et al., 2020). The large surface area of porous Au NPs can contribute to enhanced anti IAV activity compared to nonporous Au NPs. Gallic acid-modified gold nanoparticles exhibit high resistance to HSV. G-Au NPs inhibited viral attachment and penetration to vero cells and were found to be less cytotoxic than acyclovir (Halder et al., 2018). Au NPs exhibit anti-foot and mouth disease virus (FMDV) activity (Rafiei et al., 2015). Compared to chemical drugs, these nanoparticles prove to be a more effective viricidal agent and moreover do not give rise to any strains of drug resistant viruses.

They are also excellent candidates for delivering various drugs. HA-AuNP/IFNα complex for the treatment of hepatitis C infection developed by Kwang Hahn and co-workers was found to be much more stable and efficient compared to traditional drugs used (Lee et al., 2012). HIV multiplies in cells like brain microendothrlial cells, lymphocytes, macrophages etc. The ability of gold nanoparticles to enter into these cells was demonstrated by Bayo et al. They altered raltegravir (RAL), a drug employed to fight HIV, using a thiol group that acts like a connector between RAL and the gold nanoparticle. A low concentration of RAL loaded to the gold nanoparticle was converted into an active compound exhibiting preventive action against HIV (Bayo et al., 2015, Chakravarty and Vora, 2021). Small interfering RNAs (siRNAs) used for treating dengue get easily degraded by serum nucleases and eliminated easily because of their small size and anionic nature. Conjugating them with gold nanoparticles leads to high stability and can effectively fight the dengue virus (Paul et al., 2014). Peptide triazole, an HIV inhibitor when conjugated with Au NPs, exhibited enhanced activity (Bastian et al., 2015). Bowman et al. suggest that biologically inactive small molecules can be coupled with Au NPs to create active therapeutics by demonstrating with the example of SDC 1721, an inhibitor of HIV coupled with Au NPs (Bowman et al., 2008).

The virus-inhibiting capability of Au NPs is also notable. The inhibition of fusion of HIV by Au NPs is an example (Bowman et al., 2008). This is made possible by multivalent interactions of Au NPs. Dendronized Au NPs are also highly effective (Peña et al., 2016). Sialic acid-modified Au NPs, through multivalent interactions, can prevent the influenza virus (Papp et al., 2010). They prevent viruses from being attached to the host cells and reduce the chances of drug resistance development. The antiviral activities are size dependent: 14 nm Au NPs exhibit the highest antiviral capacity (Vonnemann et al., 2014). Chiodo et al. developed highly active anti-retroviral therapy (HAART) for the treatment of HIV infection using anti-HIV prodrug candidates loaded into gold nanoparticles coated with carbohydrate. The release of anti-HIV drugs from the nanoparticle was controlled by pH and antiviral activity is achieved by preventing viral replication (Chiodo et al., 2014).

Au NPs were used to modify enzyme-linked immune solvent assay (ELISA), which resulted in amplification of the signal. H1N1 and H3N2 viruses were sensed with 500-fold higher sensitivity in comparison to the test kits (Rahin et al., 2016). Au NPs are also employed in designing biomarker platforms, because of their potential to form bioconjugates with molecules like DNA and this facilitates the evolution of easy clinical diagnosis techniques (Baptista et al., 2008). Direct detection of HCV virus was made possible with unmodified Au NPs (Shawky et al., 2010). The composite of Au NPs with zirconia nanoparticles and chitosan was employed in modifying a glassy carbon electrode (GCE) used in developing an immunosensor and it was found to be highly sensitive to hepatitis C virus (HCV) core antigen (Ma et al., 2012). MersCoV can be easily detected using Au NP-based colorimetric assay (Kim et al., 2019). Many companies are now developing easy test kits based on Au NPs for point of care tests without sending the samples to laboratories (Udugama et al., 2020). Sajjanar et al. report efficiency of peptide – Au NP-based visual sensor for the virus, which allows fast and easy detection of the virus (Sajjanar et al., 2015).

Dykman and Khelbtsov, after their detailed study on the immunological properties of Au NPs, reported that they are immunostimulatory as they enhance production of proinflammatory cytokines, and can serve as adjuvants to make vaccines more effective (Dykman and Khlebtsov, 2017). But Sekimukai et al. report the failure of Au NPs as an adjuvant to generate protective antibody and bring down eosinophilic infiltration in lungs and suggest that more research is required on Au NP-adjuvanted vaccines for Covid treatment (Sekimukai et al., 2020). Vaccines based on gold nanorods against RSV infections were discovered by Stone et al. (Stone et al., 2013).

Bai et al. have reported the antiviral potential of gold nanoclusters (NCs) formed from a large number of gold atoms to inhibit porcine reproductive and respiratory syndrome virus (PRRSV) by preventing its proliferation and protein expression. They suggested that these NCs can be employed as an antiviral substance for RNA virus infections (Bai et al., 2018). Au NCs were surface modified as histidine stabilized Au NCs (His-Au NCs) and the His-Au NCs were found to inhibit the pseudorabies virus (PRV). This indicates the scope for further development of antiviral agents by altering the surface modifications like mercaptoethane sulfonate and histidine stabilized Au NCs (MES-Au NCs) and many others for controlling viruses (Feng et al., 2018).

1.2.2.3 Zinc Oxide Nanoparticles

Zinc oxide nanoparticles are also proved to be potential candidates with significant virucidal potency. Zinc oxide tetrapods (ZnOTs) block the HSV 2 virus from entering target cells and thus prevent infections (Antoine et al., 2012). Zinc oxide tetrapod nanoparticles (ZOTEN) developed by Antoine et al. were used intravaginally in nano immunotherapy to suppress HSV 2. Its strong ability to trap the virus evidently lessened vaginal infection. It also prevents reinfection by increasing the presentation of bound virions to antigen-presenting cells (APCs) (Antoine et al., 2016). Negatively charged zinc oxide micro nano structures (ZnO-MNSs) capture virions and act as a hindrance to their entry into corneal fibroblasts targeted by HSV-1 (Gurunathan et al., 2020). Tavakoli et al. investigated the effect of ZnO-NPs coated with polyethylene glycol (PEG) on HSV 1 virus and concluded that PEGylation enhances antiviral capability and reduces the cytotoxicity of nanoparticles (Tavakoli et al., 2018). Ghaffari et al. compared the activities of ZnO NPs and PEGylated ZnO NPs and confirmed the enhancement of antiviral potential against H1N1 influenza virus by PEGylation (Ghaffari et al., 2019).

1.2.3   Polymeric Nanoparticles

Large polymers and those with branches were found to exhibit high antiviral capacities (Lee et al., 1999). Polymeric nanoparticles are colloids with a size between 10 nm and 1000 nm. Synthetic and natural polymers are used in the development of polymeric nanoparticles. Biocompatible polymers approved to be safe and sound by the World Health Organization (WHO) and the Food and Drugs Administration (FDA) are used in therapeutics and other medicinal purposes (Singh et al., 2017b).

Polymeric core-shells, micelles, dendrimers, polymeric solid nanoparticles, nanocapsules, and nanospheres are all different polymer-based nanoformulations. Polymers can be designed according to the desired properties. Micelles formed above critical micelle concentration with a hydrophilic shell and hydrophobic core are employed as carriers. Drug encapsulation in these micelles imparts more stability and solubility of drugs and they also help in a higher retention time of drugs, making them more effective (Moretton et al., 2010). Nanocapsules are polymeric nanoparticles carrying the drug in its core and nanospheres carry the drug that is embedded in its matrix or absorbed into its core (Verma et al., 2017, Singh et al., 2010). Nucleoside reverse transcriptase inhibitors (NRTIs), transported into the cytoplasm in triphosphorylated form by a nanocapsule, are an example of an application of nanocapsules (Parboosing et al., 2012). Among the polymers, organotin polymers are reported to exhibit high virucidal effects. Triethyltin and trimethyltin esters were used to derive organotin polymers exhibiting high antiviral potential (Rzaev and Sadykh-Zade 1973, Chen and Liang, 2020). Organotin compounds are well known for anti-tumour actions and their antiviral capabilities have been explored recently.

The longer time periods for which these polymeric nanocarriers can be retained in the blood stream and circulate in blood without being filtered out through the kidneys easily and their better performance compared to other chemical antiviral drugs are key factors which facilitate the use of polymeric materials as antiviral agents. Their larger molecular weight, the condense structure that enable better binding of target and polymer, little resistance offered by cells to polymers, flexible structure of polymers, the improved inhibitory performance attained on changing subunits of polymers etc. have attracted greater interest in polymeric nanoparticles. The viricidal capacity of anti-tumour polymers was demonstrated and this was attributed due to the blocking of replication of viral DNA (Roner et al., 2011). The nucleic acid polymers (DNA) were also found to possess antiviral capabilities to prevent infections before and after entry of the virus into host cells (Wranke and Wedemeyer, 2016).

Polymer drug conjugates (formed with a polymer and a drug) also display excellent antiviral capacity. Conjugate formed with polyethylene glycol and α2A was observed to be efficacious against HCV (Chen et al., 2014). Poly(phenylene ethynylene) (PPE) polymers exhibit significant antiviral, antibacterial, and antifungal attributes. The usually used antibacterial agents like cationic-conjugated polyelectrolytes (CPE) based on PPE exhibit significant antiviral potential. Both CPE and oligo-phenylene ethynylenes (OPE) polymers were assessed for their antiviral effects and they were found to possess excellent antiviral potential (Wang et al., 2011).

The application of polymers as antiviral coatings is increasing. The development of polymeric nanoparticles carrying acyclovir led to a rise in the oral-bio availability as well as the activity of the drug. Polymers also act as carriers of the antiviral drug. The larger solubility and retention time and improved uptake of drugs by the targeted cells contribute to its increased demand and potential applications (Chun et al., 2018). In some polymeric nanocarriers, the potential to release drugs at a specific site is increased by varying factors like pH, using heat or employing a magnetic field, leading to the reduction of toxic effects and drug degradation (Ratemi, 2018). These nanocarriers have also helped to increase the penetrating potential of certain drugs.

Dendrimers are branched nanostructures and their structural features make them the best choice for antiviral effects and also drug encapsulation purposes for therapeutic applications. Vivagel is a dendrimer well known for its antiviral capacities against HIV and HSV (Milovanovic, 2017). Polyanionic carbosilane dendrimers (PCDs) which hinder viral entry and prevent sexually transmitted infections is also an example (Telwatte et al., 2011). Anionic groups, peptides, and carbohydrates are used to functionalize them. The micelles formed using dendrimers to encapsule anti-HCV drugs resulted in increased solubility, reduced toxicity, and helped in maintaining pH required for proper action of the drug (Lancelot et al., 2017). Looking into the measures to enhance the action of dendrimers, the dendrimers combined with tenofovir and maraviroc by Daniel et al. were reported to be helpful in preventing the sexual transmission of HIV-1(Sepúlveda et al., 2015)]. This combination was found to be highly efficient against viral infection.

1.2.4 OTHER FUNCTIONAL NANOPARTICLES

1.2.4.1 Mesoporous Silicon Nanoparticles

Mesoporous silicon nanoparticles, which exhibit low cytotoxicity and high biocompatibility and with a porous structure, were employed in antiviral drug delivery (Chen and Liang, 2020). The drug loaded in these mesoporous structures can be discharged in a constrained manner. These nanoparticles can be employed as intravaginal microbicides against diseases like genital herpes etc. The efficiency of these particles to inhibit HIV, RSP etc. was also evaluated (Osminkina et al., 2014). The nonspecific Si NPs can reduce viral infections due to their porous structure. The study on antiviral mechanisms of Si NPs revealed that the drastic changes on the surface of the virus resulting from being treated with Si NPs and caused changes in their behaviour. ML336, an inhibitor developed against the Venezuelan equine encephalitis virus (VEEV) and which can be used as a bio terrorism agent, is highly unstable. Lipid-coated mesoporous Si NPs (LC-MSNs) improved the stability of ML366 (LaBauve et al., 2018).

Different nanoparticles are being investigated for their abilities to act against pathogens in various ways. Viral infections can be prevented by the RNA interference (RNAi) method, where a nanoparticle mimics the role of the cellular RNA-induced silencing complex (RISC) mechanism facilitating cleavage of the target RNA (Zhang et al., 2014, Wang et al., 2012). HCV was treated using a nanozyme by cleaving the HCV RNA. This nanozyme is stable, nontoxic, and can be easily developed and is thus the best candidate for therapeutic applications (Wang et al., 2012, Chen and Liang, 2020).

Investigations on mechanisms to reduce viral replication so as to develop broad-spectrum antiviral agents led to new strategies. Modified drug delivery nanosystems to reduce cellular cholesterol are an example (Pollock et al., 2010). This helped in reducing HIV, HCV, and HBV infections and pretreatment of cells by suppressing cholesterol levels also reduced the rate of infection. This suggested that viral activity can be reduced by reducing virus-related cholesterol which can be employed as an antiviral strategy.

1.2.4.2 Lipid Nanoparticles

Lipid nanoparticles are also employed as drug carriers. Lipid nanoparticles are highly effective when compared to free drugs (Milovanovic et al., 2017). When compared to the polymers employed in drug delivery, lipid carriers are more biodegradable, nontoxic, and can be fabricated by easy and cost-effective methods (Puri et al., 2009).

Triglycerides, fatty acids like bee wax, lecithins etc. with small amounts of surfactants and cosolvents are the main lipids employed in drug delivery (Attama et al., 2012).

Liposomes formed by dispersion of phospholipids in water are vesicular structures where the drug is dispersed within an aqueous core. They are capable of delivering hydrophilic and hydrophobic drugs. Possessing advantages like protection of drugs from gastrointestinal degradation and capability for controlled drug delivery, they are not widely used because of drawbacks like low drug-loading capacities, physical instability issues etc. (Li et al., 2018, He et al., 2019). They are also employed as adjuvants in vaccines, as they enhance the immunity (Perrie et al., 2008).

Stable solid lipid nanoparticles (SLNs) provide protection to the drug inside, and have the ability to release the same in a controlled manner, meanwhile carrying large amounts of drug in it and being capable of targeted drug delivery. They are employed as an alternative for conventional colloidal nanoparticles like micelles, polymer nanoparticles etc, combining their advantages and eliminating drawbacks. SLNs can be synthesized in an economic and simple way (Singh et al., 2017b). Commonly used SLNs include partial glycerides, steroids, fatty acids, triglycerides, and waxes (Chakravarty and Vora, 2021). Nanostructured lipid carriers (NLCs) with better loading capacity and stability are known as second generation SLNs. Nano emulsions and nano suspensions are two other lipid-based nanoformulations. Albumin polymers are used to develop protein nanoparticles which are employed as carriers for drugs for treating cytomegalovirus infections(Milovanovic et al., 2017).

Recent developments in nanotechnology have resulted in the discovery of different functional nanomaterials exhibiting antiviral effects. Recently developed microcarriers for Zika virus antigenic peptides (Ortega-Berlanga et al., 2020), dengue virus-inhibiting curcumin-based nano emulsion (Nabila et al., 2020), nickel oxide nanostructures (NONS) counteracting cucumber mosaic virus (CMV) (Derbalah and Elsharkawy, 2019), and zinc oxide nano particle- (ZnO-NPs) derived drugs inhibiting H1N1 influenza virus (Ghaffari et al., 2019) are few among them. Electrostatic coupling with anionic poly (amino acid)-based block copolymers were used to yield antiviral amphipathic α−helical peptides (positively charged) that are antiviral peptide nanocomplexes, and were reported to be efficient in inhibiting HCV and HIV viruses (Zhang et al., 2013a).

Nanoparticles exhibit advanced virus targeting and inhibiting strategies when compared to the chemical drugs and other available methods. They are less toxic with least side effects when compared to existing practices. This has contributed to the increased attention on nanomaterials for antiviral applications.

1.3 ANTIVIRAL MECHANISM OF FUNCTIONAL NANOPARTICLES

The invasion of viruses into the body followed by its replication using the internal mechanism of the cells leads to the development of viral infections. This process involves six steps: attachment of virus on host cell, penetration of virus into the cell, uncoating of the genetic material, then replication, assembling of new virions, and finally the release of newly synthesized virions to infect the adjacent cells. Antiviral materials inhibit any of these steps to reduce and then eliminate the infection. They mainly target the stages like the initial viral entry stage, penetration, or budding.

Now, looking into various mechanisms exhibited by the antiviral nanoparticles, the best way is to inactivate the virus. Some of the nanoparticles alter the surface structure and protein of the virus, leading to their inactivation.

The main mechanism employed in preventing infections is by hindering attachment of pathogen to the host cell and saving it from being infected. The nanoparticles mimicking the target for viral attachment is another strategy used. The anti-HIV action of Ag NPs through their binding to envelope glycoprotein Gp120 of HIV and preventing its binding to the host cell is an example (Lara et al., 2010a). Nanoparticles exhibiting this mechanism can be used as wide spectrum antiviral agents to prevent infections. The low cytotoxicity exhibited by them also makes them the best choice for preventing viral infections (Cagno et al., 2018).

The penetration of pathogens can be prevented by altering the surface membrane and protein structures. These blockings developed between viruses and host cells are also highly effective in preventing infections. The replication of the virus inside after penetration can be prevented by inhibiting the synthesis of enzymes required for replication. The prevention of budding and removal of offspring viruses produced can lead to a reduction in infection. Metal nanoparticles are the best suited candidates for blocking the replication process. The prevention of entry of progeny virus to adjacent cells is found to be inhibited by nanoparticles by blocking release of neuraminidase enzyme that is used in cleavage of bonding between the progeny virus and host cell. Thus, the release of progeny is hindered leading to inhibition of the progression of infection.

Collectively it can be concluded that the main antiviral mechanisms of nanoparticles include interaction with the surface proteins of viruses, competitive inhibition by binding to host cell receptors, inhibition of penetration, inactivation of viruses before host cell invasion, blocking replication, blocking the release and development of progeny viruses etc. The different antiviral mechanisms exhibited by nanoparticles are shown in Figure 1.2.

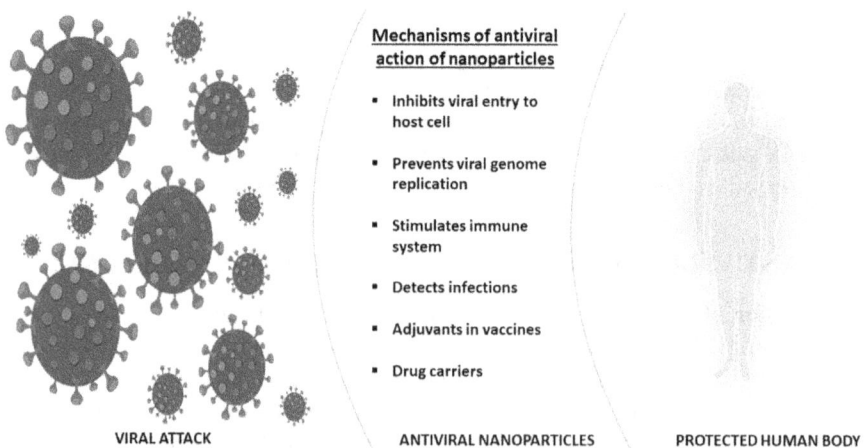

Mechanisms of antiviral action of nanoparticles

- Inhibits viral entry to host cell
- Prevents viral genome replication
- Stimulates immune system
- Detects infections
- Adjuvants in vaccines
- Drug carriers

VIRAL ATTACK   ANTIVIRAL NANOPARTICLES   PROTECTED HUMAN BODY

FIGURE 1.2 Mechanisms of viral inhibition by nanoparticles

1.4 CONCLUSION

The capacity of various nanoparticles in counteracting viral pathogens is examined in the chapter. The nanoparticles commonly employed as antiviral agents are explored and discussed. The advanced inhibitory effect of surface modified and functionalised nanoparticles is also highlighted. The ability of nanoparticles to inhibit viral binding to host cells, prevent replication of viral genomes, as efficient drug carriers that can penetrate barriers, increase the efficiency of drugs carried, as adjuvants for vaccines, as detection agents that make easy detection of infection, to stimulate immune system, entrap and destroy pathogens makes them promising candidates for developing antiviral agents. More research work in the field of progressing nanotheranostics is an urgent necessity to bring out excellent nanoparticle candidates for fighting pathogens, when viral infections continue to threaten the world, in spite of all developments.

REFERENCES

Aasi, A., Aghaei, S.M., Moore, M.D. and Panchapakesan, B., 2020. Pt-, Rh-, Ru-, and Cu-single-wall carbon nanotubes are exceptional candidates for design of anti-viral surfaces: A theoretical study. *International Journal of Molecular Sciences*, *21*(15), p.5211.

Alghrair, Z.K., Fernig, D.G. and Ebrahimi, B., 2019. Enhanced inhibition of influenza virus infection by peptide–noble-metal nanoparticle conjugates. *Beilstein Journal of Nanotechnology*, *10*(1), pp.1038–1047.

Andrade, L.M., Cox, L., Versiani, A.F. and da Fonseca, F.G., 2017. A growing world of small things: A brief review on the nanostructured vaccines. *Future Virology*, *12*(12), pp.767–779.

Antoine, T.E., Hadigal, S.R., Yakoub, A.M., Mishra, Y.K., Bhattacharya, P., Haddad, C., Valyi-Nagy, T., Adelung, R., Prabhakar, B.S. and Shukla, D., 2016. Intravaginal zinc oxide tetrapod nanoparticles as novel immunoprotective agents against genital herpes. *Journal of Immunology*, *196*(11), pp.4566–4575.

Antoine, T.E., Mishra, Y.K., Trigilio, J., Tiwari, V., Adelung, R. and Shukla, D., 2012. Prophylactic, therapeutic and neutralizing effects of zinc oxide tetrapod structures against herpes simplex virus type-2 infection. *Antiviral Research*, *96*(3), pp.363–375.

Attama, A.A., Momoh, M.A. and Builders, P.F., 2012. Lipid nanoparticulate drug delivery systems: A revolution in dosage form design and development. *Recent Advances in Novel Drug Carrier Systems*, *5*, pp.107–140.

Bai, Y., Zhou, Y., Liu, H., Fang, L., Liang, J. and Xiao, S., 2018. Glutathione-stabilized fluorescent gold nanoclusters vary in their influences on the proliferation of pseudorabies virus and porcine reproductive and respiratory syndrome virus. *ACS Applied Nano Materials*, *1*(2), pp.969–976.

Bakry, R., Vallant, R.M., Najam-ul-Haq, M., Rainer, M., Szabo, Z., Huck, C.W. and Bonn, G.K., 2007. Medicinal applications of fullerenes. *International Journal of Nanomedicine*, *2*(4), p.639.

Baptista, P., Pereira, E., Eaton, P., Doria, G., Miranda, A., Gomes, I., Quaresma, P. and Franco, R., 2008. Gold nanoparticles for the development of clinical diagnosis methods. *Analytical and Bioanalytical Chemistry*, *391*(3), pp.943–950.

Baram-Pinto, D., Shukla, S., Perkas, N., Gedanken, A. and Sarid, R., 2009. Inhibition of herpes simplex virus type 1 infection by silver nanoparticles capped with mercaptoethane sulfonate. *Bioconjugate Chemistry*, *20*(8), pp.1497–1502.

Barras, A., Pagneux, Q., Sane, F., Wang, Q., Boukherroub, R., Hober, D. and Szunerits, S., 2016. High efficiency of functional carbon nanodots as entry inhibitors of herpes simplex virus type 1. *ACS Applied Materials and Interfaces*, *8*(14), pp.9004–9013.

Bastian, A.R., Nangarlia, A., Bailey, L.D., Holmes, A., Sundaram, R.V.K., Ang, C., Moreira, D.R., Freedman, K., Duffy, C., Contarino, M. and Abrams, C., 2015. Mechanism of multivalent nanoparticle encounter with HIV-1 for potency enhancement of peptide triazole virus inactivation. *Journal of Biological Chemistry*, *290*(1), pp.529–543.

Bayo, J., Dalvi, M.P. and Martinez, E.D., 2015. Successful strategies in the discovery of small-molecule epigenetic modulators with anticancer potential. *Future Medicinal Chemistry*, *7*(16), pp.2243–2261.

Bowman, M.C., Ballard, T.E., Ackerson, C.J., Feldheim, D.L., Margolis, D.M. and Melander, C., 2008. Inhibition of HIV fusion with multivalent gold nanoparticles. *Journal of the American Chemical Society*, *130*(22), pp.6896–6897.

Cagno, V., Andreozzi, P., D'Alicarnasso, M., Silva, P.J., Mueller, M., Galloux, M., Le Goffic, R., Jones, S.T., Vallino, M., Hodek, J. and Weber, J., 2018. Broad-spectrum non-toxic antiviral nanoparticles with a virucidal inhibition mechanism. *Nature Materials*, *17*(2), pp.195–203.

Cao, C., Gontard, L.C., Thuy Tram, L.L., Wolff, A. and Bang, D.D., 2011. Dual enlargement of gold nanoparticles: From mechanism to scanometric detection of pathogenic bacteria. *Small*, *7*(12), pp.1701–1708.

Caygill, R.L., Blair, G.E. and Millner, P.A., 2010. A review on viral biosensors to detect human pathogens. *Analytica Chimica Acta*, *681*(1–2), pp.8–15.

Chakravarty, M. and Vora, A., 2021. Nanotechnology-based antiviral therapeutics. *Drug Delivery and Translational Research*, *11*(3), pp.748–787.

Chen, F., Yao, Y., Lin, H., Hu, Z., Hu, W., Zang, Z. and Tang, X., 2018. Synthesis of CuInZnS quantum dots for cell labelling applications. *Ceramics International*, *44*, pp.S34–S37.

Chen, H., Zheng, X., Nicholas, J., Humes, S.T., Loeb, J.C., Robinson, S.E., Bisesi, J.H., Das, D., Saleh, N.B., Castleman, W.L. and Lednicky, J.A., 2017. Single-walled carbon nanotubes modulate pulmonary immune responses and increase pandemic influenza A virus titers in mice. *Virology Journal*, *14*(1), pp.1–15.

Chen, L. and Liang, J., 2020. An overview of functional nanoparticles as novel emerging antiviral therapeutic agents. *Materials Science and Engineering: Part C*, *112*, p.110924.

Chen, L., Zhang, X., Zhou, G., Xiang, X., Ji, X., Zheng, Z., He, Z. and Wang, H., 2012. Simultaneous determination of human enterovirus 71 and coxsackievirus B3 by dual-color quantum dots and homogeneous immunoassay. *Analytical Chemistry*, *84*(7), pp.3200–3207.

Chen, N., Zheng, Y., Yin, J., Li, X. and Zheng, C., 2013. Inhibitory effects of silver nanoparticles against adenovirus type 3 in vitro. *Journal of Virological Methods*, *193*(2), pp.470–477.

Chen, X., Chen, X., Chen, W., Ma, X., Huang, J. and Chen, R., 2014. Extended peginterferon alfa-2a (Pegasys) therapy in Chinese patients with HBeAg-negative chronic hepatitis B. *Journal of Medical Virology*, *86*(10), pp.1705–1713.

Chen, Y.N., Hsueh, Y.H., Hsieh, C.T., Tzou, D.Y. and Chang, P.L., 2016. Antiviral activity of graphene–silver nanocomposites against non-enveloped and enveloped viruses. *International Journal of Environmental Research and Public Health*, *13*(4), p.430.

Chiodo, F., Marradi, M., Calvo, J., Yuste, E. and Penadés, S., 2014. Glycosystems in nanotechnology: Gold glyconanoparticles as carrier for anti-HIV prodrugs. *Beilstein Journal of Organic Chemistry*, *10*(1), pp.1339–1346.

Chun, H., Yeom, M., Kim, H.O., Lim, J.W., Na, W., Park, G., Park, C., Kang, A., Yun, D., Kim, J. and Song, D., 2018. Efficient antiviral co-delivery using polymersomes by controlling the surface density of cell-targeting groups for influenza A virus treatment. *Polymer Chemistry*, *9*(16), pp.2116–2123.

Daaboul, G.G., Yurt, A., Zhang, X., Hwang, G.M., Goldberg, B.B. and Unlu, M.S., 2010. High-throughput detection and sizing of individual low-index nanoparticles and viruses for pathogen identification. *Nano Letters*, *10*(11), pp.4727–4731.

Deokar, A.R., Nagvenkar, A.P., Kalt, I., Shani, L., Yeshurun, Y., Gedanken, A. and Sarid, R., 2017. Graphene-based "hot plate" for the capture and destruction of the herpes simplex virus type 1. *Bioconjugate Chemistry*, *28*(4), pp.1115–1122.

Derbalah, A.S.H. and Elsharkawy, M.M., 2019. A new strategy to control cucumber mosaic virus using fabricated NiO-nanostructures. *Journal of Biotechnology*, *306*, pp.134–141.

Dey, P., Bergmann, T., Cuellar-Camacho, J.L., Ehrmann, S., Chowdhury, M.S., Zhang, M., Dahmani, I., Haag, R. and Azab, W., 2018. Multivalent flexible nanogels exhibit broad-spectrum antiviral activity by blocking virus entry. *ACS Nano*, *12*(7), pp.6429–6442.

Domingo, E., 2010. Mechanisms of viral emergence. *Veterinary Research*, *41*(6), p.38.

Du, T., Cai, K., Han, H., Fang, L., Liang, J. and Xiao, S., 2015. Probing the interactions of CdTe quantum dots with pseudorabies virus. *Scientific Reports*, *5*(1), pp.1–10.

Du, X., Xiao, R., Fu, H., Yuan, Z., Zhang, W., Yin, L., He, C., Li, C., Zhou, J., Liu, G. and Shu, G., 2019. Hypericin-loaded graphene oxide protects ducks against a novel duck reovirus. *Materials Science and Engineering: Part C*, *105*, p.110052.

Dykman, L.A. and Khlebtsov, N.G., 2017. Immunological properties of gold nanoparticles. *Chemical Science*, *8*(3), pp.1719–1735.

Elechiguerra, J.L., Burt, J.L., Morones, J.R., Camacho-Bragado, A., Gao, X., Lara, H.H. and Yacaman, M.J., 2005. Interaction of silver nanoparticles with HIV-1. *Journal of Nanobiotechnology*, *3*(1), pp.1–10.

Ezzati Nazhad Dolatabadi, J., Omidi, Y. and Losic, D., 2011. Carbon nanotubes as an advanced drug and gene delivery nanosystem. *Current Nanoscience*, *7*(3), pp.297–314.

Falanga, A., Vitiello, M.T., Cantisani, M., Tarallo, R., Guarnieri, D., Mignogna, E., Netti, P., Pedone, C., Galdiero, M. and Galdiero, S., 2011. A peptide derived from herpes simplex virus type 1 glycoprotein H: Membrane translocation and applications to the delivery of quantum dots. *Nanomedicine: Nanotechnology, Biology and Medicine*, *7*(6), pp.925–934.

Fayaz, A.M., Ao, Z., Girilal, M., Chen, L., Xiao, X., Kalaichelvan, P.T. and Yao, X., 2012. Inactivation of microbial infectiousness by silver nanoparticles-coated condom: A new approach to inhibit HIV-and HSV-transmitted infection. *International Journal of Nanomedicine*, *7*, p.5007.

Feng, C., Fang, P., Zhou, Y., Liu, L., Fang, L., Xiao, S. and Liang, J., 2018. Different effects of His-Au NCs and MES-Au NCs on the propagation of pseudorabies virus. *Global Challenges*, *2*(8), p.1800030.

Fouad, G.I., 2021. A proposed insight into the anti-viral potential of metallic nanoparticles against novel coronavirus disease-19 (COVID-19). *Bulletin of the National Research Centre*, *45*(1), pp.1–22.

Galdiero, S., Falanga, A., Vitiello, M., Cantisani, M., Marra, V. and Galdiero, M., 2011. Silver nanoparticles as potential antiviral agents. *Molecules*, *16*(10), pp.8894–8918.

Ghaffari, H., Tavakoli, A., Moradi, A., Tabarraei, A., Bokharaei-Salim, F., Zahmatkeshan, M., Farahmand, M., Javanmard, D., Kiani, S.J., Esghaei, M. and Pirhajati-Mahabadi, V., 2019. Inhibition of H1N1 influenza virus infection by zinc oxide nanoparticles: Another emerging application of nanomedicine. *Journal of Biomedical Science*, *26*(1), pp.1–10.

Grover, N., Douaisi, M.P., Borkar, I.V., Lee, L., Dinu, C.Z., Kane, R.S. and Dordick, J.S., 2013. Perhydrolase-nanotube paint composites with sporicidal and antiviral activity. *Applied Microbiology and Biotechnology*, *97*(19), pp.8813–8821.

Gurunathan, S., Qasim, M., Choi, Y., Do, J.T., Park, C., Hong, K., Kim, J.H. and Song, H., 2020. Antiviral potential of nanoparticles—Can nanoparticles fight against coronaviruses? *Nanomaterials*, *10*(9), p.1645.

Haggag, E.G., Elshamy, A.M., Rabeh, M.A., Gabr, N.M., Salem, M., Youssif, K.A., Samir, A., Muhsinah, A.B., Alsayari, A. and Abdelmohsen, U.R., 2019. Antiviral potential of green synthesized silver nanoparticles of Lampranthuscoccineus and Malephora lutea. *International Journal of Nanomedicine, 14*, p.6217.

Halder, A., Das, S., Ojha, D., Chattopadhyay, D. and Mukherjee, A., 2018. Highly monodispersed gold nanoparticles synthesis and inhibition of herpes simplex virus infections. *Materials Science and Engineering: Part C, 89*, pp.413–421.

Hallaj-Nezhadia, S., Lotfıpour, F. and Dass, C.R., 2010. Delivery of nanoparticulate drug delivery systems via the intravenous route for cancer gene therapy. *Die Pharmazie-an International Journal of Pharmaceutical Sciences, 65*(12), pp.855–859.

Hang, X., Peng, H., Song, H., Qi, Z., Miao, X. and Xu, W., 2015. Antiviral activity of cuprous oxide nanoparticles against hepatitis C virus in vitro. *Journal of Virological Methods, 222*, pp.150–157.

He, H., Lu, Y., Qi, J., Zhu, Q., Chen, Z. and Wu, W., 2019. Adapting liposomes for oral drug delivery. *Acta Pharmaceuticasinica B, 9*(1), pp.36–48.

Huang, S., Gu, J., Ye, J., Fang, B., Wan, S., Wang, C., Ashraf, U., Li, Q., Wang, X., Shao, L. and Song, Y., 2019. Benzoxazine Monomer Derived Carbon Dots as a Broad-Spectrum Agent to Block viral infectivity.. *Journal of colloid and Interface Science, 542*, 198–206.

Huang, X. and El-Sayed, M.A., 2010. Gold nanoparticles: Optical properties and implementations in cancer diagnosis and photothermal therapy. *Journal of Advanced Research, 1*(1), pp.13–28.

Iannazzo, D., Mazzaglia, A., Scala, A., Pistone, A., Galvagno, S., Lanza, M., Riccucci, C., Ingo, G.M., Colao, I., Sciortino, M.T. and Valle, F., 2014. β-cyclodextrin-grafted on multiwalled carbon nanotubes as versatile nanoplatform for entrapment of guanine-based drugs. *Colloids and Surfaces, Part B: Biointerfaces, 123*, pp.264–270.

Iannazzo, D., Pistone, A., Galvagno, S., Ferro, S., De Luca, L., Monforte, A.M., Da Ros, T., Hadad, C., Prato, M. and Pannecouque, C., 2015. Synthesis and anti-HIV activity of carboxylated and drug-conjugated multi-walled carbon nanotubes. *Carbon, 82*, pp.548–561.

Iannazzo, D., Pistone, A., Ferro, S., De Luca, L., Monforte, A.M., Romeo, R., Buemi, M.R. and Pannecouque, C., 2018. Graphene quantum dots based systems as HIV inhibitors. *Bioconjugate Chemistry, 29*(9), pp.3084–3093.

Ingle, A.P., Duran, N. and Rai, M., 2014. Bioactivity, mechanism of action, and cytotoxicity of copper-based nanoparticles: A review. *Applied Microbiology and Biotechnology, 98*(3), pp.1001–1009.

Khandelwal, N., Kaur, G., Chaubey, K.K., Singh, P., Sharma, S., Tiwari, A., Singh, S.V. and Kumar, N., 2014. Silver nanoparticles impair Peste des petits ruminants virus replication. *Virus Research, 190*, pp.1–7.

Kim, H., Park, M., Hwang, J., Kim, J.H., Chung, D.R., Lee, K.S. and Kang, M., 2019. Development of label-free colorimetric assay for MERS-CoV using gold nanoparticles. *ACS Sensors, 4*(5), pp.1306–1312.

Kim, J., Yeom, M., Lee, T., Kim, H.O., Na, W., Kang, A., Lim, J.W., Park, G., Park, C., Song, D. and Haam, S., 2020. Porous gold nanoparticles for attenuating infectivity of influenza A virus. *Journal of Nanobiotechnology, 18*(1), pp.1–11.

Kotelnikova, R.A., Bogdanov, G.N., Frog, E.C., Kotelnikov, A.I., Shtolko, V.N., Romanova, V.S., Andreev, S.M., Kushch, A.A., Fedorova, N.E., Medzhidova, A.A. and Miller, G.G., 2003. Nanobionicsof pharmacologically active derivatives of fullerene C 60. *Journal of Nanoparticle Research, 5*(5), pp.561–566.

Kumar, R., Dhanawat, M., Kumar, S., Singh, B.N., Pandit, J.K. and Sinha, V.R., 2014. Carbon nanotubes: A potential concept for drug delivery applications. *Recent Patents on Drug Delivery and Formulation, 8*(1), pp.12–26.

Kuppusamy, P., Ichwan, S.J., Parine, N.R., Yusoff, M.M., Maniam, G.P. and Govindan, N., 2015. Intracellular biosynthesis of Au and Ag nanoparticles using ethanolic extract of Brassica oleracea L. and studies on their physicochemical and biological properties. *Journal of Environmental Sciences*, 29, pp.151–157.

LaBauve, A.E., Rinker, T.E., Noureddine, A., Serda, R.E., Howe, J.Y., Sherman, M.B., Rasley, A., Brinker, C.J., Sasaki, D.Y. and Negrete, O.A., 2018. Lipid-coated mesoporous silica nanoparticles for the delivery of the ML336 antiviral to inhibit encephalitic Alphavirus infection. *Scientific Reports*, 8(1), pp.1–13.

Lancelot, A., Clavería-Gimeno, R., Velázquez-Campoy, A., Abian, O., Serrano, J.L. and Sierra, T., 2017. Nanostructures based on ammonium-terminated amphiphilic Janus dendrimers as camptothecin carriers with antiviral activity. *European Polymer Journal*, 90, pp.136–149.

Lara, H.H., Ayala-Nuñez, N.V., Ixtepan-Turrent, L. and Rodriguez-Padilla, C., 2010a. Mode of antiviral action of silver nanoparticles against HIV-1. *Journal of Nanobiotechnology*, 8(1), pp.1–10.

Lara, H.H., Ixtepan-Turrent, L., Garza-Treviño, E.N. and Rodriguez-Padilla, C., 2010b. PVP-coated silver nanoparticles block the transmission of cell-free and cell-associated HIV-1 in human cervical culture. *Journal of Nanobiotechnology*, 8(1), pp.1–11.

Lee, J., Ahmed, S.R., Oh, S., Kim, J., Suzuki, T., Parmar, K., Park, S.S., Lee, J. and Park, E.Y., 2015. A plasmon-assisted fluoro-immunoassay using gold nanoparticle-decorated carbon nanotubes for monitoring the influenza virus. *Biosensors and Bioelectronics*, 64, pp.311–317.

Lee, K.J., Angulo, A., Ghazal, P. and Janda, K.D., 1999. Soluble-polymer supported synthesis of a prostanoid library: Identification of antiviral activity. *Organic Letters*, 1(11), pp.1859–1862.

Lee, M.Y., Yang, J.A., Jung, H.S., Beack, S., Choi, J.E., Hur, W., Koo, H., Kim, K., Yoon, S.K. and Hahn, S.K., 2012. Hyaluronic acid–gold nanoparticle/interferon α complex for targeted treatment of hepatitis C virus infection. *ACS Nano*, 6(11), pp.9522–9531.

Lin, Z., Li, Y., Guo, M., Xu, T., Wang, C., Zhao, M., Wang, H., Chen, T. and Zhu, B., 2017. The inhibition of H1N1 influenza virus-induced apoptosis by silver nanoparticles functionalized with zanamivir. *RSC Advances*, 7(2), pp.742–750.

Li, T., Cipolla, D., Rades, T. and Boyd, B.J., 2018. Drug nanocrystallisation within liposomes. *Journal of Controlled Release*, 288, pp.96–110.

Liu, H., Bai, Y., Zhou, Y., Feng, C., Liu, L., Fang, L., Liang, J. and Xiao, S., 2017. Blue and cyan fluorescent carbon dots: One-pot synthesis, selective cell imaging and their antiviral activity. *RSC Advances*, 7(45), pp.28016–28023.

Liu, Y., 2018. *Multifunctional Gold Nanostars for Cancer Theranostics*. Springer Theses.

Łoczechin, A., Séron, K., Barras, A., Giovanelli, E., Belouzard, S., Chen, Y.T., Metzler-Nolte, N., Boukherroub, R., Dubuisson, J. and Szunerits, S., 2019. Functional carbon quantum dots as medical countermeasures to human coronavirus. *ACS Applied Materials and Interfaces*, 11(46), pp.42964–42974.

Lu, L., Sun, R.W.Y., Chen, R., Hui, C.K., Ho, C.M., Luk, J.M., Lau, G.K. and Che, C.M., 2008. Silver nanoparticles inhibit hepatitis B virus replication. *Antiviral Therapy*, 13(2), pp.253–262.

Lü, S., Wu, Y. and Liu, H., 2017. Silver nanoparticles synthesized using Eucommia ulmoides bark and their antibacterial efficacy. *Materials Letters*, 196, pp.217–220.

Ma, C., Xie, G., Zhang, W., Liang, M., Liu, B. and Xiang, H., 2012. Label-free sandwich type of immunosensor for hepatitis C virus core antigen based on the use of gold nanoparticles on a nanostructured metal oxide surface. *Microchimica Acta*, 178(3), pp.331–340.

Madamsetty, V.S., Mukherjee, A. and Mukherjee, S., 2019. Recent trends of the bio-inspired nanoparticles in cancer theranostics. *Frontiers in Pharmacology*, 10, p.1264.

Malik, P., Gulati, N., Malik, R.K. and Nagaich, U., 2013. Carbon nanotubes, quantum dots and dendrimers as potential nanodevices for nanotechnology drug delivery systems. *International Journal of Pharmaceutical Sciences and Nanotechnology*, 6(3), pp.2113–2124.

Michalet, X., Pinaud, F.F., Bentolila, L.A., Tsay, J.M., Doose, S.J.J.L., Li, J.J., Sundaresan, G., Wu, A.M., Gambhir, S.S. and Weiss, S., 2005. Quantum dots for live cells, in vivo imaging, and diagnostics. *Science*, 307(5709), pp.538–544.

Milovanovic, M., Arsenijevic, A., Milovanovic, J., Kanjevac, T. and Arsenijevic, N., 2017. Nanoparticles in antiviral therapy. In Alexandru Mihai Grumezescu ed. : *Antimicrobial Nanoarchitectonics* (pp.383–410). Elsevier.

Morens, D.M., Folkers, G.K. and Fauci, A.S., 2004. The challenge of emerging and re-emerging infectious diseases. *Nature*, 430(6996), pp.242–249.

Moretton, M.A., Glisoni, R.J., Chiappetta, D.A. and Sosnik, A., 2010. Molecular implications in the nanoencapsulation of the anti-tuberculosis drug rifampicin within flower-like polymeric micelles. *Colloids and Surfaces, Part B: Biointerfaces*, 79(2), pp.467–479.

Mori, Y., Ono, T., Miyahira, Y., Nguyen, V.Q., Matsui, T. and Ishihara, M., 2013. Antiviral activity of silver nanoparticle/chitosan composites against H1N1 influenza A virus. *Nanoscale Research Letters*, 8(1), pp.1–6.

Mostafavi, S.T., Mehrnia, M.R. and Rashidi, A.M., 2009. Preparation of nanofilter from carbon nanotubes for application in virus removal from water. *Desalination*, 238(1–3), pp.271–280.

Nabila, N., Suada, N.K., Denis, D., Yohan, B., Adi, A.C., Veterini, A.S., Anindya, A.L., Sasmono, R.T. and Rachmawati, H., 2020. Antiviral action of curcumin encapsulated in nanoemulsion against four serotypes of dengue virus. *Pharmaceutical Nanotechnology*, 8(1), pp.54–62.

NavaniethaKrishnaraj, R., Chandran, S., Pal, P. and Berchmans, S., 2014. Investigations on the antiretroviral activity of carbon nanotubes using computational molecular approach. *Combinatorial Chemistry and High Throughput Screening*, 17(6), pp.531–535.

Neto, A.J.P. and Fileti, E.E., 2018. Elucidating the amphiphilic character of graphene oxide. *Physical Chemistry Chemical Physics*, 20(14), pp.9507–9515.

Nierengarten, I. and Nierengarten, J.F., 2014. Fullerene sugar balls: A new class of biologically active fullerene derivatives. *Chemistry–An Asian Journal*, 9(6), pp.1436–1444.

Nitsche, C., Holloway, S., Schirmeister, T. and Klein, C.D., 2014. Biochemistry and medicinal chemistry of the dengue virus protease. *Chemical Reviews*, 114(22), pp.11348–11381.

Orłowski, P., Kowalczyk, A., Tomaszewska, E., Ranoszek-Soliwoda, K., Węgrzyn, A., Grzesiak, J., Celichowski, G., Grobelny, J., Eriksson, K. and Krzyzowska, M., 2018. Antiviral activity of tannic acid modified silver nanoparticles: Potential to activate immune response in herpes genitalis. *Viruses*, 10(10), p.524.

Ortega-Berlanga, B., Hernández-Adame, L., del Angel-Olarte, C., Aguilar, F., Rosales-Mendoza, S. and Palestino, G., 2020. Optical and biological evaluation of upconverting Gd_2O_3: Tb^{3+}/Er^{3+} particles as microcarriers of a Zika virus antigenic peptide. *Chemical Engineering Journal*, 385, p.123414.

Osminkina, L.A., Timoshenko, V.Y., Shilovsky, I.P., Kornilaeva, G.V., Shevchenko, S.N., Gongalsky, M.B., Tamarov, K.P., Abramchuk, S.S., Nikiforov, V.N., Khaitov, M.R. and Karamov, E.V., 2014. Porous silicon nanoparticles as scavengers of hazardous viruses. *Journal of Nanoparticle Research*, 16(6), pp.1–10.

Pan, H., Zhang, P., Gao, D., Zhang, Y., Li, P., Liu, L., Wang, C., Wang, H., Ma, Y. and Cai, L., 2014. Noninvasive visualization of respiratory viral infection using bioorthogonal conjugated near-infrared-emitting quantum dots. *ACS Nano*, 8(6), pp.5468–5477.

Papp, I., Sieben, C., Ludwig, K., Roskamp, M., Böttcher, C., Schlecht, S., Herrmann, A. and Haag, R., 2010. Inhibition of influenza virus infection by multivalent sialic-acid-functionalized gold nanoparticles. *Small*, *6*(24), pp.2900–2906.

Parboosing, R., Maguire, G.E., Govender, P. and Kruger, H.G., 2012. Nanotechnology and the treatment of HIV infection. *Viruses*, *4*(4), pp.488–520.

Paul, A.M., Shi, Y., Acharya, D., Douglas, J.R., Cooley, A., Anderson, J.F., Huang, F. and Bai, F., 2014. Delivery of antiviral small interfering RNA with gold nanoparticles inhibits dengue virus infection in vitro. *The Journal of General Virology*, *95*(8), p.1712.

Peña-González, C.E., García-Broncano, P., Ottaviani, M.F., Cangiotti, M., Fattori, A., Hierro-Oliva, M., González-Martín, M.L., Pérez-Serrano, J., Gómez, R., Muñoz-Fernández, M.Á. and Sánchez-Nieves, J., 2016. Dendronized anionic gold nanoparticles: Synthesis, characterization, and antiviral activity. *Chemistry–A European Journal*, *22*(9), pp.2987–2999.

Perrie, Y., Mohammed, A.R., Kirby, D.J., McNeil, S.E. and Bramwell, V.W., 2008. Vaccine adjuvant systems: Enhancing the efficacy of sub-unit protein antigens. *International Journal of Pharmaceutics*, *364*(2), pp.272–280.

Pokhrel, R., Sompornpisut, P., Chapagain, P., Olson, B., Gerstman, B. and Pandey, R.B., 2018. Domain rearrangement and denaturation in Ebola virus protein VP40. *AIP Advances*, *8*(12), p.125129.

Pollock, S., Nichita, N.B., Böhmer, A., Radulescu, C., Dwek, R.A. and Zitzmann, N., 2010. Polyunsaturated liposomes are antiviral against hepatitis B and C viruses and HIV by decreasing cholesterol levels in infected cells. *Proceedings of the National Academy of Sciences*, *107*(40), pp.17176–17181.

Pradhan, B., Guha, D., Murmu, K.C., Sur, A., Ray, P., Das, D. and Aich, P., 2017. Comparative efficacy analysis of anti-microbial peptides, LL-37 and indolicidin upon conjugation with CNT, in human monocytes. *Journal of Nanobiotechnology*, *15*(1), pp.1–16.

Puri, A., Loomis, K., Smith, B., Lee, J.H., Yavlovich, A., Heldman, E. and Blumenthal, R., 2009. Lipid-based nanoparticles as pharmaceutical drug carriers: From concepts to clinic. *Critical Reviews™ in Therapeutic Drug Carrier Systems*, *26*(6), pp. 523–80.

Rafiei, S., Rezatofighi, S.E., Ardakani, M.R. and Rastegarzadeh, S., 2015. Gold nanoparticles impair foot-and-mouth disease virus replication. *IEEE Transactions on Nanobioscience*, *15*(1), pp.34–40.

Rahin, A.S., Jeonghyo, K., Tetsuro, S. and Jaebeom, L., 2016. *Detection of Influenza Virus Using Peroxidase-mimic of Gold Nanoparticles*, Wiley.

Ratemi, E., 2018. pH-responsive polymers for drug delivery applications. *Stimuli Responsive Polymeric Nanocarriers for Drug Delivery Applications*, *1*, pp.121–141.

Reina, G., Peng, S., Jacquemin, L., Andrade, A.F. and Bianco, A., 2020. Hard nanomaterials in time of viral pandemics. *ACS Nano*, *14*(8), pp.9364–9388.

Rogers, J.V., Parkinson, C.V., Choi, Y.W., Speshock, J.L. and Hussain, S.M., 2008. A preliminary assessment of silver nanoparticle inhibition of monkeypox virus plaque formation. *Nanoscale Research Letters*, *3*(4), pp.129–133.

Roner, M.R., Carraher Jr, C.E., Shahi, K. and Barot, G., 2011. Antiviral activity of metal-containing polymers—Organotin and cisplatin-like polymers. *Materials*, *4*(6), pp.991–1012.

Russo, E., Gaglianone, N., Baldassari, S., Parodi, B., Cafaggi, S., Zibana, C., Donalisio, M., Cagno, V., Lembo, D. and Caviglioli, G., 2014. Preparation, characterization and in vitro antiviral activity evaluation of foscarnet-chitosan nanoparticles. *Colloids and Surfaces, Part B: Biointerfaces*, *118*, pp.117–125.

Rzaev, Z.M. and Sadykh-Zade, S.I., 1973. Radical copolymerization of maleic anhydride with organotin acrylates. In: Mihail C. Roco ed. *Journal of Polymer Science: Polymer*

Symposia (Vol. 42, No. 2, pp.541–552). New York: Wiley Subscription Services, Inc., A Wiley Company.

Sajjanar, B., Kakodia, B., Bisht, D., Saxena, S., Singh, A.K., Joshi, V., Tiwari, A.K. and Kumar, S., 2015. Peptide-activated gold nanoparticles for selective visual sensing of virus. *Journal of Nanoparticle Research*, *17*(5), pp.1–9.

Sametband, M., Kalt, I., Gedanken, A. and Sarid, R., 2014. Herpes simplex virus type-1 attachment inhibition by functionalized graphene oxide. *ACS Applied Materials and Interfaces*, *6*(2), pp.1228–1235.

Sekimukai, H., Iwata-Yoshikawa, N., Fukushi, S., Tani, H., Kataoka, M., Suzuki, T., Hasegawa, H., Niikura, K., Arai, K. and Nagata, N., 2020. Gold nanoparticle-adjuvanted S protein induces a strong antigen-specific IgG response against severe acute respiratory syndrome-related coronavirus infection, but fails to induce protective antibodies and limit eosinophilic infiltration in lungs. *Microbiology and Immunology*, *64*(1), pp.33–51.

Sengupta, J. and Hussain, C.M., 2020. Carbon nanomaterials to combat virus: A perspective in view of COVID-19. *Carbon Trends*, p.100019.

Sepúlveda-Crespo, D., Sánchez-Rodríguez, J., Serramía, M.J., Gómez, R., De La Mata, F.J., Jiménez, J.L. and Muñoz-Fernández, M.Á., 2015. Triple combination of carbosilane dendrimers, tenofovir and maraviroc as potential microbicide to prevent HIV-1 sexual transmission. *Nanomedicine*, *10*(6), pp.899–914.

Shao, W., Arghya, P., Yiyong, M., Rodes, L. and Prakash, S., 2013. Carbon nanotubes for use in medicine: Potentials and limitations. *Syntheses and Applications of Carbon Nanotubes and their Composites*, *13*, pp.285–311.

Shawky, S.M., Bald, D. and Azzazy, H.M., 2010. Direct detection of unamplified hepatitis C virus RNA using unmodified gold nanoparticles. *Clinical Biochemistry*, *43*(13–14), pp.1163–1168.

Sinclair, T.R., van den Hengel, S.K., Raza, B.G., Rutjes, S.A., de RodaHusman, A.M., Peijnenburg, W.J., Roesink, H.E.D. and de Vos, W.M., 2021. Surface chemistry-dependent antiviral activity of silver nanoparticles. *Nanotechnology*, *32*(36), p.365101.

Singh, A., Garg, G. and Sharma, P.K., 2010. Nanospheres: A novel approach for targeted drug delivery system. *International Journal of Pharmaceutical Sciences Review and Research*, *5*(3), pp.84–88.

Singh, A. and Sahoo, S.K., 2014. Magnetic nanoparticles: A novel platform for cancer theranostics. *Drug Discovery Today*, *19*(4), pp.474–481.

Singh, A.V., Hosseinidoust, Z., Park, B.W., Yasa, O. and Sitti, M., 2017a. Microemulsion-based soft bacteria-driven microswimmers for active cargo delivery. *ACS Nano*, *11*(10), pp.9759–9769.

Singh, L., Kruger, H.G., Maguire, G.E., Govender, T. and Parboosing, R., 2017b. The role of nanotechnology in the treatment of viral infections. *Therapeutic Advances in Infectious Disease*, *4*(4), pp.105–131.

Sofy, A.R., Hmed, A.A., Abd El Haliem, N.F., Zein, M.A.E. and Elshaarawy, R.F., 2019. Polyphosphonium-oligochitosans decorated with nanosilver as new prospective inhibitors for common human enteric viruses. *Carbohydrate Polymers*, *226*, p.115261.

Song, Z., Wang, X., Zhu, G., Nian, Q., Zhou, H., Yang, D., Qin, C. and Tang, R., 2015. Virus capture and destruction by label-free graphene oxide for detection and disinfection applications. *Small*, *11*(9–10), pp.1171–1176.

Speshock, J.L., Murdock, R.C., Braydich-Stolle, L.K., Schrand, A.M. and Hussain, S.M., 2010. Interaction of silver nanoparticles with Tacaribe virus. *Journal of Nanobiotechnology*, *8*(1), pp.1–9.

Sreekanth, T.V.M., Nagajyothi, P.C., Muthuraman, P., Enkhtaivan, G., Vattikuti, S.V.P., Tettey, C.O., Kim, D.H., Shim, J. and Yoo, K., 2018. Ultra-sonication-assisted silver nanoparticles using panax ginseng root extract and their anti-cancer and antiviral activities. *Journal of Photochemistry and Photobiology, Part B: Biology, 188*, pp.6–11.

Stone, J.W., Thornburg, N.J., Blum, D.L., Kuhn, S.J., Wright, D.W. and Crowe Jr, J.E., 2013. Gold nanorod vaccine for respiratory syncytial virus. *Nanotechnology, 24*(29), p.295102.

Sun, L., Singh, A.K., Vig, K., Pillai, S.R. and Singh, S.R., 2008. Silver nanoparticles inhibit replication of respiratory syncytial virus. *Journal of Biomedical Nanotechnology, 4*(2), pp.149–158.

Sun, R.W.Y., Chen, R., Chung, N.P.Y., Ho, C.M., Lin, C.L.S. and Che, C.M., 2005. Silver nanoparticles fabricated in Hepes buffer exhibit cytoprotective activities toward HIV-1 infected cells. *Chemical Communications, 40*, pp.5059–5061.

Szymańska, E., Orłowski, P., Winnicka, K.,Tomaszewska, E., Bąska, P., Celichowski, G., Grobelny, J., Basa, A. and Krzyżowska, M., 2018. Multifunctional tannic acid/silver nanoparticle-based mucoadhesive hydrogel for improved local treatment of HSV infection: In vitro and in vivo studies. *International Journal of Molecular Sciences, 19*(2), p.387.

Tam, P.D., Van Hieu, N., Chien, N.D., Le, A.T. and Tuan, M.A., 2009. DNA sensor development based on multi-wall carbon nanotubes for label-free influenza virus (type A) detection. *Journal of Immunological Methods, 350*(1–2), pp.118–124.

Tavakoli, A., Ataei-Pirkooh, A., Mm Sadeghi, G., Bokharaei-Salim, F., Sahrapour, P., Kiani, S.J., Moghoofei, M., Farahmand, M., Javanmard, D. and Monavari, S.H., 2018. Polyethylene glycol-coated zinc oxide nanoparticle: An efficient nanoweapon to fight against herpes simplex virus type 1. *Nanomedicine, 13*(21), pp.2675–2690.

Telwatte, S., Moore, K., Johnson, A., Tyssen, D., Sterjovski, J., Aldunate, M., Gorry, P.R., Ramsland, P.A., Lewis, G.R., Paull, J.R. and Sonza, S., 2011. Virucidal activity of the dendrimer microbicide SPL7013 against HIV-1. *Antiviral Research, 90*(3), pp.195–199.

Ting, D., Dong, N., Fang, L., Lu, J., Bi, J., Xiao, S. and Han, H., 2018. Multisite inhibitors for enteric coronavirus: Antiviral cationic carbon dots based on curcumin. *ACS Applied Nano Materials, 1*(10), pp.5451–5459.

Tong, T., Hu, H., Zhou, J., Deng, S., Zhang, X., Tang, W., Fang, L., Xiao, S. and Liang, J., 2020. Glycyrrhizic-acid-based carbon dots with high antiviral activity by multisite inhibition mechanisms. *Small, 16*(13), p.1906206.

Trefry, J.C. and Wooley, D.P., 2013. Silver nanoparticles inhibit vaccinia virus infection by preventing viral entry through a macropinocytosis-dependent mechanism. *Journal of Biomedical Nanotechnology, 9*(9), pp.1624–1635.

Udugama, B., Kadhiresan, P., Kozlowski, H.N., Malekjahani, A., Osborne, M., Li, V.Y., Chen, H., Mubareka, S., Gubbay, J.B. and Chan, W.C., 2020. Diagnosing COVID-19: The disease and tools for detection. *ACS Nano, 14*(4), pp.3822–3835.

Verma, G., Rajagopalan, M.D., Valluru, R. and Sridhar, K.A., 2017. Nanoparticles: A novel approach to target tumors. In: *Nano-and Microscale Drug Delivery Systems* (pp.113–129), Editor: Alexandru Grumezescu. Elsevier.

Versiani, A.F., Astigarraga, R.G., Rocha, E.S., Barboza, A.P.M., Kroon, E.G., Rachid, M.A., Souza, D.G., Ladeira, L.O., Barbosa-Stancioli, E.F., Jorio, A. and Da Fonseca, F.G., 2017. Multi-walled carbon nanotubes functionalized with recombinant dengue virus 3 envelope proteins induce significant and specific immune responses in mice. *Journal of Nanobiotechnology, 15*(1), pp.1–13.

Vonnemann, J., Sieben, C., Wolff, C., Ludwig, K., Böttcher, C., Herrmann, A. and Haag, R., 2014. Virus inhibition induced by polyvalent nanoparticles of different sizes. *Nanoscale, 6*(4), pp.2353–2360.

Wang, Y., Canady, T.D., Zhou, Z., Tang, Y., Price, D.N., Bear, D.G., Chi, E.Y., Schanze, K.S. and Whitten, D.G., 2011. Cationic phenylene ethynylene polymers and oligomers exhibit efficient antiviral activity. *ACS Applied Materials and Interfaces*, *3*(7), pp.2209–2214.

Wang, Z., Liu, H., Yang, S.H., Wang, T., Liu, C. and Cao, Y.C., 2012. Nanoparticle-based artificial RNA silencing machinery for antiviral therapy. *Proceedings of the National Academy of Sciences of the United States of America*, *109*(31), pp.12387–12392.

Weiss, C., Carriere, M., Fusco, L., Capua, I., Regla-Nava, J.A., Pasquali, M., Scott, J.A., Vitale, F., Unal, M.A., Mattevi, C. and Bedognetti, D., 2020. Toward nanotechnology-enabled approaches against the COVID-19 pandemic. *ACS Nano*, *14*(6), pp.6383–6406.

White, K.M., Abreu Jr, P., Wang, H., De Jesus, P.D., Manicassamy, B., García-Sastre, A., Chanda, S.K., DeVita, R.J. and Shaw, M.L., 2018. Broad spectrum inhibitor of influenza A and B viruses targeting the viral nucleoprotein. *ACS Infectious Diseases*, *4*(2), pp.146–157.

Wranke, A. and Wedemeyer, H., 2016. Antiviral therapy of hepatitis delta virus infection—Progress and challenges towards cure. *Current Opinion in Virology*, *20*, pp.112–118.

Wu, F., Yuan, H., Zhou, C., Mao, M., Liu, Q., Shen, H., Cen, Y., Qin, Z., Ma, L. and Li, L.S., 2016. Multiplexed detection of influenza A virus subtype H5 and H9 via quantum dot-based immunoassay. *Biosensors and Bioelectronics*, *77*, pp.464–470.

Yang, X.X., Li, C.M., Li, Y.F., Wang, J. and Huang, C.Z., 2017. Synergistic antiviral effect of curcumin functionalized graphene oxide against respiratory syncytial virus infection. *Nanoscale*, *9*(41), pp.16086–16092.

Yang, X.X., Li, C.M. and Huang, C.Z., 2016. Curcumin modified silver nanoparticles for highly efficient inhibition of respiratory syncytial virus infection. *Nanoscale*, *8*(5), pp.3040–3048.

Yeh, Y.T., Gulino, K., Zhang, Y., Sabestien, A., Chou, T.W., Zhou, B., Lin, Z., Albert, I., Lu, H., Swaminathan, V. and Ghedin, E., 2020. A rapid and label-free platform for virus capture and identification from clinical samples. *Proceedings of the National Academy of Sciences of the United States of America*, *117*(2), pp.895–901.

Ye, S., Shao, K., Li, Z., Guo, N., Zuo, Y., Li, Q., Lu, Z., Chen, L., He, Q. and Han, H., 2015. Antiviral activity of graphene oxide: How sharp edged structure and charge matter. *ACS Applied Materials and Interfaces*, *7*(38), pp.21571–21579.

Yong, K., Wang, Y., Roy, I., Rui, H., Swihart, M.T., Law, W., Kwak, S.K., Ye, L., Liu, J., Mahajan, S.D. and Reynolds, J.L., 2012. Preparation of quantum dot/drug nanoparticle formulations for traceable targeted delivery and therapy. *Theranostics*, *2*(7), p.681.

Yousaf, M., Huang, H., Li, P., Wang, C. and Yang, Y., 2017. Fluorine functionalized graphene quantum dots as inhibitor against hIAPP amyloid aggregation. *ACS Chemical Neuroscience*, *8*(6), pp.1368–1377.

Zhang, J., Mulvenon, A., Makarov, E., Wagoner, J., Knibbe, J., Kim, J.O., Osna, N., Bronich, T.K. and Poluektova, L.Y., 2013a. Antiviral peptide nanocomplexes as a potential therapeutic modality for HIV/HCV co-infection. *Biomaterials*, *34*(15), pp.3846–3857.

Zhang, X., Zhao, P., Wu, K., Zhang, Y., Peng, M. and Liu, Z., 2014. Compositional equivalency of RNAi-mediated virus-resistant transgenic soybean and its nontransgenic counterpart. *Journal of Agricultural and Food Chemistry*, *62*(19), pp.4475–4479.

Zhang, Y.B., Kanungo, M., Ho, A.J., Freimuth, P., Van Der Lelie, D., Chen, M., Khamis, S.M., Datta, S.S., Johnson, A.C., Misewich, J.A. and Wong, S.S., 2007. Functionalized carbon nanotubes for detecting viral proteins. *Nano Letters*, *7*(10), pp.3086–3091.

Zhang, Y., Ke, X., Zheng, Z., Zhang, C., Zhang, Z., Zhang, F., Hu, Q., He, Z. and Wang, H., 2013b. Encapsulating quantum dots into enveloped virus in living cells for tracking virus infection. *ACS Nano*, *7*(5), pp.3896–3904.

2 An Overview of Applications of Nanotechnology in the Antimicrobial Field

Sartaj Ahmad Mir, Vipin Shrotriya,
Md. Amzad Hossain, and M Burhanuz Zaman

CONTENTS

2.1 INTRODUCTION

Microorganisms in short known as microbes include organisms like bacteria, fungi (yeasts and molds), algae, viruses, etc., and have dimensions of the order of few microns. Due to their smaller size dimensions, these organisms are invisible to the naked eye. The broad classification of microbes includes prokaryotes and eukaryotes. Prokaryotes are primitive microbes that lack a distinct nucleus and other cell organelles due to the absence of internal membranes. Almost all bacteria are prokaryotic and are classified among the best-known prokaryotes. A prokaryotic cell

DOI: 10.1201/9781003243175-2

is enclosed by a cell membrane made of phospholipids. Besides the presence of a double-stranded deoxyribonucleic acid chromosome, the prokaryotic cell contains ribosomes swimming in the cytoplasm that are responsible for protein synthesis. The eukaryotic cell is the advanced version of the prokaryotic cell and is characterized by the presence of a well-defined nucleus with a proper nuclear membrane. The eukaryotic cell has proper cell organelles including mitochondria, endoplasmic reticulum, Golgi apparatus, etc. As humans, we are associated with microbes since we are born. Some among these are beneficial to the human body whereas most are detrimental, causing severe illnesses and in some cases even death. The disease-causing microbes are known as pathogens. Some of the human diseases or conditions caused by microbes are malaria, the common cold, chicken pox, tuberculosis, etc. Presently, the disastrous worldwide pandemic caused because of COVID-19 is among the worst microbial infections. It is a well-known fact that whenever humans suffer, they always find a way out. With the advent of medical science, scientists developed several antibiotics that were used to treat microbial infections [1]. As time progressed microbes have developed multi-drug resistance and advanced versions of the microbes with different strains have evolved [1–2]. For instance, the breakthrough in the field of antibiotics is the discovery of penicillin from Penicillin Rubens by Alexander Fleming. Penicillin was successfully used to treat many deadly infections of that time such as strep throat, gonorrhoea, pneumonia, etc. The success of penicillin in treating such deadly infections resulted in an overwhelming consumption of penicillin. The uncontrolled consumption of penicillin resulted in the development of new penicillin-resistant strains. The most resistant strains included Staphylococci. To tackle this issue, methicillin, a semisynthetic penicillin variety, was developed and used successfully. The same problem was faced with methicillin after some years of its clinical consumption where new methicillin-resistant strains of Staphylococcus aureus (MRSA) evolved and the antibiotic was no longer effective. This happens with most antibiotics: after a period of their consumption new microbial strains evolve that are antibiotic resistant. Thus, treating microbial infections by antibiotics has always been a challenge. According to the report put forward by the Centers for Disease Control and Prevention (CDC) in the US, it is estimated that more than two million people get infected and about 23000 people die per annum globally because of antibiotic-resistant pathogens [3]. Alternative strategies are thus required and therefore intensive work is going on in the field globally. A promising new strategy of a microbicidal approach has been introduced in the biomedical field where scientists use medical devices containing antimicrobial nanostructures [4]. Nanoparticles (NPs) have the potential to serve as novel antimicrobial agents having less chance of developing microbial resistance. Such devices have received significant attention in both academia and the pharmaceutical industry. So far, the nanostructures utilized as antimicrobial agents mostly include metal and metal oxide nanostructures [4–8]. Among various metal oxide nanostructures (ZnO, AgO, CuO etc.), ZnO has shown exceptional antimicrobial activity [8]. Metal nanoparticles working as antimicrobial agents are leading at the front. Copper, silver, gold, and other metal nanoparticles have been explored as antimicrobial agents and the antimicrobial activity exhibited is quite impressive [4].

In this chapter the author has penned down the antimicrobial applications of the nanoparticles, in particular metal and metal oxide nanoparticles. Factors influencing the antimicrobial activity of the nanostructures are discussed and the mechanisms involved are elaborated.

2.2   MICROBIAL RESISTANCE TO ANTIBIOTICS

With the gloomed success against microbial infections by the development of anti-biotics, the US Surgeon General William H. Stewart in the late 1960s stated that "it is time to close the book on infectious diseases and declare war against pesti-lence won when the success of antimicrobial therapies for controlling infectious diseases was at large." The resistance development to antibiotics proved the state-ment inaccurate. This is the reason that microbial infections are the second leading cause of death globally [9]. Whenever humans or animals consume antibiotics for the treatment of microbial infections, there is a strong chance for the development of antibiotic resistance [10]. Thus, to tackle this issue it is essential to identify the mechanism behind this biochemical resistance development. As the resistance is developed by the microbes, it depends on the microbial makeup (biochemical and genetic aspects). Several other factors decide the development of microbial resistance including antibiotic nature, target site, etc. Microbes develop resistance against antibiotics generally by inactivating those using enzymes. The enzymes modify or degrade the antibiotics via several processes including hydrolysis, group transfer, or redox mechanism. During the hydrolysis process, the enzymes break the weak bonds of amides and esters of the antibiotics thus making the antibiotic molecules inactive [11].

Several enzymes (the transferase group) inactivate the antibiotics by attaching the functional groups via chemical substitution to the outer boundary of the antibiotic molecules. This modification of the antibiotic molecules results in their inactiveness because modified molecules do not have suitable sites to bind to the target sites [12]. As far as redox process-based antibiotic inactivation is concerned the mechanism is rarely found. Oxidation of tetracycline by the TetX enzyme present in the conjuga-tive transposon of B. Fragilis is one of the best examples where this mechanism is followed [13]. The resistance mechanism involved in the microbial kingdom is sche-matically shown in **Figure 2.1.**

2.3   NANOMATERIALS AS ALTERNATIVES TO ANTIBIOTICS TO TACKLE MICROBIAL RESISTANCE

The issue of that faced by humans due to the developed antibiotic-resistant microbial strains means that permanent and long-term solutions are required. Nanomaterials are proven to be better alternatives and are presently serving as a solution to the problem. The nanoparticles as per studies are used as broad-spectrum antibiotics. It has been found that for the development of microbial resistance to the nanoparticles, simultaneous mutations need to arise, but that is less likely to occur and hence there are fewer chances of the development of microbial resistance to nanoparticles [14].

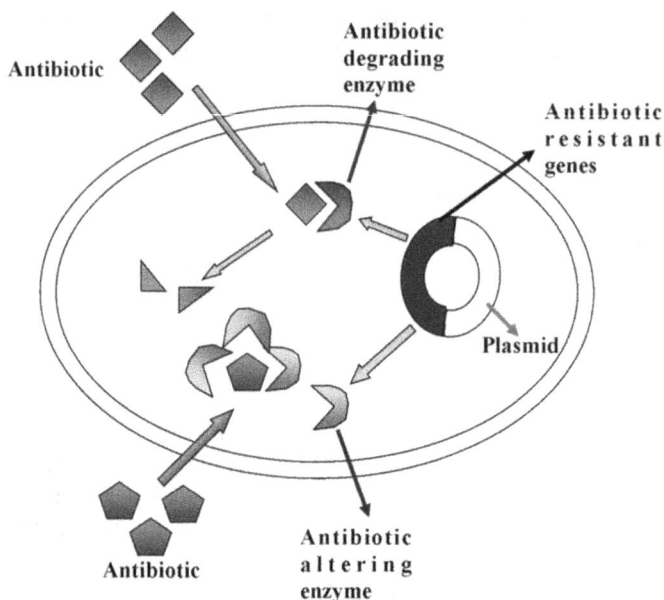

FIGURE 2.1   Mechanism of antimicrobial resistance.

2.4   FACTORS INFLUENCING THE ANTIMICROBIAL ACTIVITY OF NANOSTRUCTURES

There are two entities involved as far as the antimicrobial applications of the nanoparticles are concerned: the nanoparticles and the microbes. Thus, both nanoparticle properties, as well as the microbe cell structure, have a great role to play in antimicrobial activity.

2.4.1   MICROBES' CELL STRUCTURE

As far as the antimicrobial applications of nanoparticles, the cell wall and membranes are important defensive barriers for bacterial resistance to environmental toxicity [15]. In the case of bacteria, based on the cell wall structure bacteria are classified as Gram-positive and Gram-negative. The cell structures of the two bacterial categories are shown in **Figure 2.2**. The cell wall in the case of the Gram-positive contains a thick layer of peptidoglycan whereas the layer is thin in the case of Gram-negative bacteria. Peptidoglycan is a polymer containing sugars and amino acids that play an important structural role in the bacterial cell wall, providing structural strength, and counteracting cytoplasmic osmotic pressure. In addition to the peptidoglycan layer, an outer membrane of lipopolysaccharide is there for Gram-negative bacteria and is termed "periplasm." This arrangement of layers in the case of Gram-negative bacteria generally facilitates the ions' movement across the cell wall. The thicker wall of peptidoglycan has teichoic and teteichuronic acids that are covalently attached and

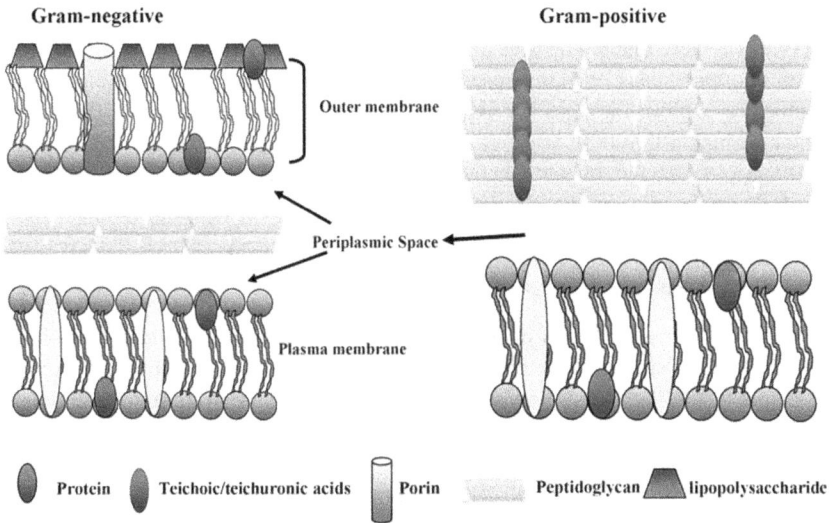

FIGURE 2.2   Bacterial cell wall structure.

hinder cell wall damage. This therefore makes the nanoparticles less toxic to Gram-positive bacteria [16]. Thus, because of the inbuilt cell structure, Gram-negative bacteria are more prone to the toxicity of the nanoparticles. Moreover, the lipopolysaccharide coating being negatively charged makes Gram-negative cells more susceptible to the nanoparticles generating positive ions [16]. This factor results in higher intake transport of the nanoparticles that causes intracellular damage. The bacterial cell wall is negative in both cases (Gram-positive and Gram-negative); however, studies showed that E. Coli (Gram-negative) is more negative than S. aureus (Gram-positive) and hence more prone to nanoparticle toxicity [17]. This is because the Gram-negative cell wall is populated with a mosaic of negative surface domains rather than a continuous layer that results in a potential binding of nanoparticles and is hence more prone to the toxicity of nanostructures. Proof of this electrostatic interaction is provided by the study in the case of reactive oxygen species (ROS). It was found that RROS-like hydroxyl radicals were not allowed to easily pass through the negatively charged cell membrane. The repulsion between the ROS and cell membrane provided valid proof of electrostatic involvement. There is an exception to this electrostatic interaction in the case of heavy metals and the theory of electrostatic interaction is not valid. This behaviour is found in the case of heavy metal resistant bacteria where the bacteria cell was not influenced by heavy metallic nanoparticles. In this respect the most frequently studied microbes include *P aeruginosa* and *E coli*. The studies revealed the co-existence of resistance to numerous heavy metals and antibiotic classes [18, 19]. There are several other studies where the same types of bacteria behave differently to identical nanoparticles. For instance, consider an example from the literature where TiO$_2$ nanoparticles were explored as antibacterial agents against *E coli* and *C metallidurans* (Gram-negative bacteria). The results were quite surprising; the nanoparticles were effective for only *E coli* [18]. The same observations were made when these bacteria were exposed to the toxicity of another type of nanoparticles [19]. This observation found in the case of *C metallidurans* led scientists to explore the possible explanation. Further studies made in the field led to the conclusion that the two large plasmids (pMol-28 and pMol-30) conferred the metal resistance shown by the bacteria. Transcriptomatic analysis revealed that these two plasmids were responsible for the upregulation of 83 and 143 genes [20].

2.4.2 NANOPARTICLE PROPERTIES

There are certain parameters of the nanoparticles that influence their microbicidal activity. Some of such parameters include nanoparticles' dimension, surface charge, and shape. A detailed discussion is penned down under a separate subheading below.

2.4.2.1 Nanoparticle Dimensions

The antimicrobial activity is directly proportional to the surface-to-volume ratio of the nanostructures. The nanostructures with a high surface-to-volume ratio are expected to have high antimicrobial activity and are suitable for surface-related applications [21, 22]. This ratio will be high if the nanoparticles are of lower dimensions. At lower dimensions the physical and chemical properties of the nanoparticles get modified – that also affects the antimicrobial ability. Smaller-sized nanostructures are associated with a large specific surface area. It is a general statement that the larger the specific surface area, the higher the antimicrobial activity of the nanostructures. This fact regarding smaller nanostructures with a high specific surface area makes nanoparticles more detrimental to microbial life. In the context of the effect of nanoparticle size on antimicrobial activity, various researchers examined the situation and came to the same conclusion. For instance, in the case of Ag-decorated TiO2 nanorods, N Esfandiari et al. reported that the antimicrobial activity depended on the size characteristics of the Ag-TiO2 coating and was highest in the case where the TiO2 nanorods were decorated with the smallest sized (20 nm) Ag nanoparticles [23]. Osonga et al. while studying the antimicrobial activity of Ag and Au nanoparticles observed that smaller Ag nanoparticles (9 nm) exhibited higher antimicrobial activity [24]. In some cases this hypothesis fails where larger nanostructures are more effective than smaller ones. This indicated that size alone is not the factor influencing the microbial activity.

2.4.2.2 Nanoparticle Shape

The shape is also an effective parameter that decides the activity of the nanoparticles. Possible shapes exhibited by the nanoparticles are spheres, sheets, plates, tubes, cubes, rods, and triangles [17]. The specific surface area exhibited by the nanoparticles is determined by their shape and surface area has direct proportionality with the antimicrobial activity. If we go for the geometry of the shapes, the spherical shape has the least specific surface area.

Some reports show nanocubes and nanorods are more effective. To justify the reason for this, an observation analysis of the exposed crystal facets was carried out by several researchers. According to the analysis, unstable surfaces are prone to oxygen vacancies, linking the bactericidal activity of the NPs to the stability of the planes [25]. It was reported that identical surface areas with different particle shapes behave differently because the high atomic density facet planes increase reactivity [26, 27]. There is a relation between the presence of corners, edges, or defects (increased abrasiveness) and toxicity: (i) a large area helps in better adsorption and binding of compounds, and (ii) the increase in surface defects results in enhanced surface area to volume ratio which has a direct effect on ROS generation [28].

2.5   NANOPARTICLE SURFACE CHARGE

The surface charge of the nanoparticles has a direct influence on the antimicrobial property of the nanoparticles [17]. The bacterial surfaces are mostly negative and hence as per the electrostatic interaction nanoparticles with positive surfaces would be the most effective. In this regard nanoparticles generating positive ions in the microbial broth are highly effective as per the physical interaction is concerned. The first step involved in the antimicrobial activity is the physical adsorption of the nanoparticles onto the cell wall. This adsorption will be higher if the surface charge of the nanoparticles is positive. This is because metallic nanoparticles and metallic ions are most effective in the area of an antimicrobial field. Moreover, in the case of metallic nanoparticles, the ion-releasing ability of the nanoparticles in the bacterial broth is also an important factor. For instance, let us take an example of copper and silver nanoparticles. L.A. Tamayo et al. undertook a report on how the release of Ag and Cu nanoparticles affects their antimicrobial activity. The authors observed and noted in their article that the ion-releasing tendency from nanoparticles is element dependent. They found that copper nanoparticles release copper ions more easily than silver nanoparticles do. Based on their statistical report they mentioned that copper nanoparticles release about 253 times more ions than silver nanoparticles do [29]. The higher the ability to release the ions, the larger the antibacterial ability.

2.6   METAL OXIDE NANOSTRUCTURES AS ANTIMICROBIAL AGENTS

2.6.1   COPPER OXIDE (CUO)

Due to the intrinsic antimicrobial activity exhibited by copper, semiconductor nanostructures having copper as one of their elements makes such nanomaterials suitable candidates for fabricating antimicrobial devices, bandages, ointments, etc. CuO, because of its excellent antimicrobial activity, has attracted the interest of material scientists and has led to the development of new antimicrobial ointments, antimicrobial coatings, and bandages. This material has been recognized by the US Environmental Protection Agency (EPA) as antimicrobial material [30, 31]. These nanomaterials have been used against various strains of Gram-negative and Gram-positive bacteria [32–35]. These nanoparticles can inhibit biofilm formation on medical devices. There are several reports in the literature where authors have used

CuO nanoparticles to inhibit biofilm formation. This behaviour has been reported for both Gram-negative as well as Gram-positive bacteria [36]. The microbicidal activity of the CuO depends on several physicochemical parameters like shape and the size of the nanomaterials. In one study, Y H Hsueh et al. observed that even the pH of the precursor solution determines the activity of the nanoparticles. The literature revealed high toxicity of the nanoparticles at low pH values [37]. It has been observed that at low pH values the nanoparticles penetrate effectively into the microbe cells. Yi-Huang Hsueh et al. reported and explained in detail how pH influences the antimicrobial activity of the CuO nanoparticles. The authors explored the nanoparticles against Staphylococcus aureus (S. aureus) four strains: viz. Newman, SA113, USA300, and ATCC6538 [37]. The conclusion from the study was that the releasing and penetrating ability of the Cu^{2+} ions into the cell was effective with a lower pH (4–4.5) that determined the extent of the toxicity of the CuO nanoparticle. The efficient releasing power of copper ions made the nanoparticles more toxic to the microorganisms. As the microbial activity is influenced by the shape and size of the nanostructures, various researchers have studied the antimicrobial property of CuO nanostructures having different shapes and sizes. In a report it was found that octahedral-shaped CuO nanoparticles were more effective than cube-shaped nanoparticles as far as antimicrobial activity was concerned [38]. In another study it was found that CuO nanosheets were more biocidal [39]. This higher activity of specific shaped CuO nanostructures is justified by the fact that different surface facets have different adsorption-desorption abilities towards the microorganisms [40]. Researchers provided two mechanisms that describe the antimicrobial activity of CuO nanostructures with different shapes. The first mechanism takes into account the physical interaction between the two entities (nanoparticles and the microbial cell wall). The higher the interaction, the better the activity. Differently shaped nanoparticles interact with the cell wall differently. The irregular edge-shaped nanostructures (sheets) perturb the cell wall effectively and hence exhibit better activity. Chemically it has been observed that CuO nanosheets verified a high biochemical activity during GSH oxidation. A general mechanism involves contact killing in which CuO releases copper ions which then generate reactive oxygen species thereby disrupting cellular membranes. The ROS generated causes the degradation of cellular biomolecules. There are some other reports where researchers claim that CuO nanoparticles inactivate certain cellular enzymes that are responsible for metabolic pathways. Thus, in conclusion, it is the Cu ion-releasing ability of the Cu-based nanoparticles that determines the antimicrobial activity.

2.6.2 Zinc Oxide (ZnO)

Besides applications in the engineering field, ZnO nanostructures have a good reputation in medicine. In biology and medicine, due to their anticancer [41], antimicrobial, and fungicidal activities [42, 43], anti-inflammatory activity [44, 45], ability to accelerate wound healing [46], and antidiabetic properties [47, 48] ZnO nanostructures have gained popularity. ZnO behaves as a wide spectrum antimicrobial agent and has been explored against microorganisms including Escherichia coli,

Staphylococcus aureus, Pseudomonas aeruginosa, Bacillus subtilis, and the M13 bacteriophage [49–52]. The ZnO of different morphologies (rods, needles, spheres, and platelets) influence antimicrobial activity. The shape and particle size distribution are the key parameters that decide nanoparticle uptake into cell membranes and thereby determine their action. Regarding ZnO literature, there are reports of morphology tuning including tuning the shape and size of nanostructures in order to enhance the antimicrobial activity. In a report Tamimi et al. synthesized ZnO nanorods, nanospheres, and nanoparticles and investigated the antimicrobial activity of all three types of ZnO nanostructures [53]. The authors studied the influence of zinc oxide morphology on the antimicrobial properties of tapioca starch films. The authors concluded that nanosphere-shaped ZnO particles exhibit the highest antibacterial properties. Other shapes like bowtie-, flower-, and nest-shaped ZnO particles reported in the literature were explored against E. coli and S. Aureus to check their antimicrobial activity [54]. In this study the authors observed almost no influence of shape on the antimicrobial activity of the nanostructures. Their experiments revealed that antibacterial activity is not morphology-dependent only. They conclude that differences in particle surface area, pore size, synthesis approach, and building blocks also determine antimicrobial activity of the nanostructures. The morphological tuning of ZnO by pH variation is a common method. In a report by Saliani et al., ZnO morphology was tuned by varying the pH of the precursor solution and the corresponding influence of morphology on antimicrobial activity was investigated [55]. The literature is summarized in Table 2.1 which illustrates different shaped ZnO nanostructures and their antimicrobial activity.

TABLE 2.1
Differently Shaped ZnO Nanostructures Used as Broad-Spectrum Antibiotics Reported in the Literature

Morphology	Particle size (nm)	Microbe investigated	Reference
Sphere	12	S. aureus	[56]
	15-20	Streptococcus and Serratia	[57]
	<100	E. coli	[58]
	16–60 nm	E. coli and S. aureus	[59]
Rods	Length 523 nm; diameter 47 nm	S. aureus	[60]
	Length ~2 µm; diameter ~50 nm	E. coli, S. aureus, and P. aeruginosa	[61]
Needles	Length ~2 µm; diameter 20–40 nm	*E coli, S aureus, K pneumoniae, B subtilis, B cereus, S marcescens*	[62]
Hollow tubes	Length ~500 nm	*S aureus, B subtilis E coli, and P aeruginosa*	[63]
	Length ~5 µm; thickness 59.5 nm	*S aureus and E coli*	[64]

2.7   METAL NANOSTRUCTURES AS ANTIMICROBIAL AGENTS

2.7.1   Silver (Ag)

Silver nanoparticles (Ag NPs) are proven to be outstanding microbicidal agents and can fight in vitro and in vivo bacterial infections. They have potential action against Gram-positive as well as Gram-negative bacteria [65]. Literature is flooded with articles describing the antimicrobial activity of Ag nanoparticles. This material exhibits unique properties at the nanoscale dimensions due to which Ag NPs led to the fabrication of different products like targeted drug delivery, diagnosis, detection, and imaging [66–73]. However, due to the outstanding antibacterial activity shown by Ag, NPs they have fascinated material scientists and biologists worldwide. Hence these nanoparticles have gained prominence amongst researchers and industries. The antibacterial activity made these nanoparticles most precious in medical and healthcare areas. The properties of the Ag NPs resulted in the incorporation of these nanoparticles in various medical products including cosmetics, surgical tools, dressings, and dental tools [74–76]. The antibiotic aspect of Ag NPs is related to their different mechanisms of action. The nanoparticles attack microbes in multiple structures at a time that provide them with the ability to destroy various types of bacteria. The literature reports three mechanisms that elaborate the working of Ag NPs as antimicrobial agents [77–79]. Ag NPs act at the membrane level and are adsorbed over the cell membrane from where these penetrate into the cell cytoplasm. Once the nanoparticle enters the cell cytoplasm, these get adsorbed over the inner membranes that cause membrane destabilization and damage. This results in increased membrane permeability and the induced leakage of cellular content and finally its death [80, 81]. In the second mechanism proposed by several researchers, the NPs not only can break and cross the cell membrane, but can interact with the intercellular sulphur or phosphorus groups of DNA and proteins thereby altering their structure and hence functions. This is how these nanoparticles can alter the respiratory chain where the nanoparticles interact with the thiol groups. The third mechanism proposed in parallel with the above two mechanisms involves the release of silver ions, which depending on particle size and charge, can interact with cellular components altering metabolic pathways, membranes, and even genetic material [82].

As per the reports, Ag NPs are antimicrobial agents that have the potential capability of fighting against almost 650 types of microbial infections [83]. The first report about medical applications of Ag NPs was published in 1881 in which the authors explored Ag NPs to treat eye infections in neonates. Later on, in 1901 Ag NPs were consumed as internal antisepsis. Nowadays, silver nitrate- and silver sulfadiazine-containing drugs are commonly used to treat wounds and dermal burns, and to remove warts [84]. The literature has articles that report the tuning of properties that influence the antimicrobial activity of Ag nanostructures. Zheng et al. reported the size-dependent antimicrobial activity of the nanoparticles and concluded that the activity increases appreciably when the size of the nanostructures is below 10 nm [84]. The high penetration ability across the cell membranes makes smaller nanoparticles more toxic to the microbes. Furthermore, in recent studies it was observed that the small functionalized Ag NPs severely control processes like mitochondrial electron transport, organelle integrity, phagocytosis, autophagy, and organization [85]. Casey et al. studied the size-dependent microbicidal activity of Ag NPs against E. Coli and reported that the size of the NPs has an inverse relation with the activity. The authors believed that the ion-releasing ability is the prime factor that affects antimicrobial activity. The enhanced antimicrobial activity of the NPs was explained by the Gibbs-Thomson phenomenon. A particle with increased curvature (smaller particles) will dissolute more ions [86]. Y Dong et al. fabricated different-sized spherical Ag NPs by adjusting the pH of the precursor solution. The authors used Vibrio natriegens as a model to compare the antibacterial activities of Ag NPs with different particle sizes and concluded that smaller NPs are more toxic to the microbial cell [87].

Tang et al. studied the influence of Ag nanoparticle shapes on antimicrobial activity. In their work, three shapes were analyzed including spherical, rod-shaped, and truncated triangular-shaped against E. coli bacteria. In the study, it was observed that the triangular-shaped nanoparticles were more effective followed by the spheres and finally rods. The reason for this high activity of the triangular-shaped nanoparticles was according to the authors ascribed to the highest number of the facets of the nanoparticles that caused increased surface binding, cell uptake, and finally microbial death [88]. In another report, Ag nanoparticles with different morphologies including spheres, rods, cubes, and platelets were explored against Staphylococcus aureus. The bactericidal ability was ascribed to the dissolution kinetics and therefore to the particle morphology [89].

2.7.2 GOLD (AU)

Au NPs have great potential in drug delivery platforms including antimicrobial applications. In the case of gold nanoparticles, due to their unique applications in the medical field, the literature is full of articles where the authors worked on tuning all the properties that influenced the antimicrobial activity of the nanoparticles. Modifications in shape, size, and particle surface have been performed from time to time by material scientists. There are various approaches that they use to control the size of the Ag nanoparticles, including the Brust-Schiffrin method, Turkevich method, Murphy method, Perrault method, etc. The Brust-Schiffrin method involves the use of $NaBH_4$ as the reductant in which nanoparticles as small as 2–10 nm of Ag are prepared. In the Turkevich method 1,0–20 nm particles are prepared where citrate ions are used to control the growth of the nanoparticles. The Murphy method results in the formation of 10–50 nm Au NPs and this control is governed by the chemical nature of ascorbic acid [90]. Recently in an article, J. Osonga studied the shape- and size-dependent antibacterial activity of the Ag and Au NPs. The results obtained by them indicated that the nanoparticles inhibited the growth of both Gram (+) and Gram (−) bacteria. The nanoparticles were more effective for Gram (+) bacteria [91]. S Zhu et al. reported the synthesis of Au NPs having variable particle sizes using chlorogenic acid [92]. As far as the morphology of the gold nanoparticles is concerned, different shapes have been reported in the literature. J Penders et al.

reported the synthesis of antimicrobial Au NPs of various shapes (spheres, stars, and flowers), having similar dimensions. According to the results obtained the authors concluded that Au NPs having a flower-like shape possessed the most promising non-cytotoxic mammalian cell behaviour with the greatest shape-dependent anti-bacterial activity-promising properties [93]. In another report by S Hameed et al., spheres (Au NSps), stars (Au NSts), and cubes (Au NCs) were investigated against E coli, P aeruginosa, and S aureus at lower concentrations. Au NCs were observed to be more effective bactericidal agents with a 100% inactivation rate [94].

2.8 SUMMARY

In summary, the chapter deals with the antimicrobial applications of metal and metal oxide nanostructures. The drawbacks of antibiotics were overcome by the antimi-crobial nanoparticles that tackle microbial infections effectively. The nature of the microbes greatly influences the attaching ability of the nanostructures that directly depends on electrostatic interactions. If the electrostatic forces are attractive the adhe-sion will be good and as is also the case with metal nanostructures. Metal nanostruc-tures are effective against Gram-negative bacteria: because of electrostatic attractions, the nanoparticles adhere effectively to the bacterial cell membrane. This is why metal nanostructures are more detrimental to microbes. The shape, size, and surface charge of the nanostructures largely influence microbial activity. Smaller nanoparticles due to a large surface area are more effective than bulk material. The nanoparticles with large active facets have better activity. The physical interactions are very important and constitute the first step of the antimicrobial mechanism. ZnO and Ag nanopar-ticles are currently regarded as the best antimicrobial agents at the laboratory level. These nanoparticles are now being commercialized, and used in cosmetics and other antiseptic ointments. The market demand for such products is gradually increasing.

REFERENCES

1. Davies, J., & Davies, D. Origins and evolution of antibiotic resistance. *Microbiology and Molecular Biology Reviews* (2010), 74(3), 417–433. https://doi.org/10.1128/mmbr .00016-10.
2. Fair, R.J., & Tor, Y. Antibiotics and bacterial resistance in the 21st century. *Perspectives in Medicinal Chemistry* (2014), 6. https://doi.org/10.4137/pmc.s14459.
3. CDC. *Antibiotic Resistance Threats in the United States, 2019.* Atlanta, GA: U.S. Department of Health and Human Services, CDC, 2019.
4. Erkoc, P., & Ulucan-Karnak, F. Nanotechnology-based antimicrobial and antivi-ral surface coating strategies. *Prosthesis* (2021), 3(1), 25–52. https://doi.org/10.3390/ prosthesis3010005.
5. Zaman, M.B., Poolla, R., Singh, P., & Gudipati, T. Biogenic synthesis of CuO Nanoparticles using Tamarindus indica L. and a study of their photocatalytic and antibacterial activity. *Environmental Nanotechnology, Monitoring and Management* (2020), 100346. https://doi.org/10.1016/j.enmm.2020.100346.
6. Zhang, Y., Shareena Dasari, T.P., Deng, H., & Yu, H. Antimicrobial activity of gold nanoparticles and ionic gold. *Journal of Environmental Science and Health, Part C* (2015), 33(3), 286–327. https://doi.org/10.1080/10590501.2015.1055161.

7. Heinonen, S., Nikkanen, J.-P., Laakso, J., Raulio, M., Priha, O., & Levänen, E. Bacterial growth on a superhydrophobic surface containing silver nanoparticles. *IOP Conference Series: Materials Science and Engineering* (2013), 47, 012064. https://doi.org/10.1088/1757-899x/47/1/012064.

8. Zhang, R., Liu, X., Xiong, Z., Huang, Q., Yang, X., Yan, H., Ma, J., Feng, Q., & Shen, Z. Novel micro/nanostructured TiO_2/ZnO coating with antibacterial capacity and cytocompatibility. *Ceramics International* (2018), 44(8), 9711–9719. https://doi.org/10.1016/j.ceramint.2018.02.20.

9. Spellberg, B., Guidos, R., Gilbert, D., Bradley, J., Boucher, H.W., Scheld, W.M., Bartlett, J.G., Edwards, J., & Infectious Diseases Society of America. The epidemic of antibiotic-resistant infections: A call to action for the medical community from the Infectious Diseases Society of America. *Clinical Infectious Diseases* (2008), 46(2), 155–164. https://doi.org/10.1086/524891.

10. Austin, D.J., Kristinsson, K.G., & Anderson, R.M. The relationship between the volume of antimicrobial consumption in human communities and the frequency of resistance. *Proceedings of the National Academy of Sciences of the United States of America* (1999), 96(3), 1152–1156. https://doi.org/10.1073/pnas.96.3.1152.

11. Peterson, E., & Kaur, P. Antibiotic resistance mechanisms in bacteria: Relationships Between resistance determinants of antibiotic producers, environmental bacteria, and clinical pathogens. *Frontiers in Microbiology* (2018), 9. https://doi.org/10.3389/fmicb.2018.02928.

12. Kumar, S., & Varela, M.F. Molecular mechanisms of bacterial resistance to antimicrobial agents. In: *Microbial Pathogens and Strategies for Combating Them: Science, Technology and Education*; Méndez-Vilas, A., Ed.; Badajoz: Formatex Research Center, pp. 522–534, 2013.

13. Wright, G. Bacterial resistance to antibiotics: Enzymatic degradation and modification. *Advanced Drug Delivery Reviews* (2005), 57(10), 1451–1470. https://doi.org/10.1016/j.addr.2005.04.002.

14. Huh, A.J., & Kwon, Y.J. "Nanoantibiotics": A new paradigm for treating infectious diseases using nanomaterials in the antibiotics resistant era. *Journal of Controlled Release* (2011), 156(2), 128–145. https://doi.org/10.1016/j.jconrel.2011.07.002.

15. Wang, L., Hu, C., & Shao, L. The antimicrobial activity of nanoparticles: Present situation and prospects for the future. *International Journal of Nanomedicine* (2017), 12, 1227–1249. https://doi.org/10.2147/ijn.s121956.

16. Slavin, Y.N., Asnis, J., Häfeli, U.O., & Bach, H. Metal nanoparticles: Understanding the mechanisms behind antibacterial activity. *Journal of Nanobiotechnology* (2017), 15(1). https://doi.org/10.1186/s12951-017-0308-z.

17. Sonohara, R., Muramatsu, N., Ohshima, H., & Kondo, T. Difference in surface properties between Escherichia coli and Staphylococcus aureus as revealed by electrophoretic mobility measurements. *Biophysical Chemistry* (1995), 55(3), 273–277. https://doi.org/10.1016/0301-4622(95)00004-h.

18. Simon-Deckers, A., Loo, S., Mayne-L'hermite, M., Herlin-Boime, N., Menguy, N., Reynaud, C., Gouget, B., & Carrière, M. Size-, composition- and shape-dependent toxicological impact of metal oxide nanoparticles and carbon nanotubes toward bacteria. *Environmental Science and Technology* (2009), 43(21), 8423–8429. https://doi.org/10.1021/es9016975.

19. Pignon, B., Maskrot, H., Guyot Ferreol, V., Leconte, Y., Coste, S., Gervais, M., Pouget, T., Reynaud, C., Tranchant, J., & Herlin-Boime, N. Versatility of laser pyrolysis applied to the synthesis of TiO_2 nanoparticles— Application to UV attenuation. *European Journal of Inorganic Chemistry* (2008), 2008(6), 883–889.

20. Monchy, S., Benotmane, M.A., Janssen, P., Vallaeys, T., Taghavi, S., van der Lelie, D., & Mergeay, M. Plasmids pMOL28 and pMOL30 of Cupriavidus metallidurans are

specialized in the maximal viable response to heavy metals. *Journal of Bacteriology* (2007), 189(20), 7417–7425.

21. Gudipati, T., Zaman, M.B., Singh, P., & Poolla, R. Enhanced photocatalytic activity of biogenically synthesized CuO nanostructures against xylenol orange and rhodamine b dyes. *Inorganic Chemistry Communications* (2021), 130, 108677. https://doi.org/10.1016/j.inoche.2021.108677.

22. Masrat, S., Poolla, R., Dipak, P., & Burhanuz Zaman, M. Rapid hydrothermal synthesis of highly crystalline transition metal (Mn & Fe) doped CuSe nanostructures: Applications in wastewater treatment and room temperature gas sensing. *Surfaces and Interfaces* (2021), 23, 100973. https://doi.org/doi.org/10.1016/j.surfin.2021.100973.

23. Esfandiari, N., Simchi, A., & Bagheri, R. Size tuning of Ag-decorated TiO_2 nanotube arrays for improved bactericidal capacity of orthopedic implants. *Journal of Biomedical Materials Research – Part A* (2013), 102(8), 2625–2635. https://doi.org/10.1002/jbm.a.34934.

24. Osonga, F.J., Akgul, A., Yazgan, I., Akgul, A., Eshun, G.B., Sakhaee, L., & Sadik, O.A. Size and shape-dependent antimicrobial activities of silver and gold nanoparticles: A model study as potential fungicides. *Molecules* (2020), 25(11), 2682. https://doi.org/10.3390/molecules25112682.

25. Wang, L., He, H., Yu, Y., Sun, L., Liu, S., Zhang, C., & He, L. Morphology-dependent bactericidal activities of Ag/CeO_2 catalysts against Escherichia coli. *Journal of Inorganic Biochemistry* (2014), 135, 45–53. https://doi.org/10.1016/j.jinorgbio.2014.02.0.

26. Pal, S., Tak, Y.K., & Song, J.M. Does the antibacterial activity of silver nanoparticles depend on the shape of the nanoparticle? A study of the Gram-negative bacterium Escherichia coli. *Applied and Environment Microbiology* (2007), 73(6), 1712–1720.

27. Morones, J.R., Elechiguerra, J.L., Camacho, A., Holt, K., Kouri, J.B., Ramírez, J.T., & Yacaman, M.J. The bactericidal effect of silver nanoparticles. *Nanotechnology* (2005), 16(10), 2346.

28. Stoimenov, P.K., Klinger, R.L., Marchin, G.L., & Klabunde, K.J. Metal oxide nanoparticles as bactericidal agents. *Langmuir* (2002), 18(17), 6679–6686.

29. Tamayo, L.A., Zapata, P.A., Vejar, N.D., Azócar, M.I., Gulppi, M.A., Zhou, X., Thompson, G.E., Rabagliati, F.M., & Páez, M.A. Release of silver and copper nanoparticles from polyethylene nanocomposites and their penetration into Listeria monocytogenes. *Materials Science and Engineering. Part C* (2014), 40, 24–31.

30. Wang, Y., Yang, F., Zhang, H., Zi, X., Pan, X., Chen, F., Luo, W., Li, J., Zhu, H., & Hu, Y. Cuprous oxide nanoparticles inhibit the growth and metastasis of melanoma by targeting mitochondria. *Cell Death and Disease* (2013), 4(8), e783.

31. Yang, Q., Wang, Y., Yang, Q., Gao, Y., Duan, X., Fu, Q., Chu, C., Pan, X., Cui, X., & Sun, Y. Cuprous oxide nanoparticles trigger ER stress-induced apoptosis by regulating copper trafficking and overcoming resistance to sunitinib therapy in renal cancer. *Biomaterials* (2017), 146, 72–85.

32. Grass, G., Rensing, C., & Solioz, M. Metallic copper as an antimicrobial surface. *Applied and Environment Microbiology* (2011), 77(5), 1541–1547.

33. Du, B.D., Phu, D.V., Quoc, L.A., & Hien, N.Q. Synthesis and investigation of antimicrobial activity of Cu_2O nanoparticles/zeolite. *Journal of Nanoparticles* (2017), 2017, 1.

34. Ashjari, H.R., Dorraji, M.S.S., Fakhrzadeh, V., Eslami, H., Rasoulifard, M.H., Rastgouy-Houjaghan, M., Gholizadeh, P., & Kafil, H.S. Starch-based polyurethane/CuO nanocomposite foam: Antibacterial effects for infection control. *International Journal of Biological Macromolecules* (2018), 111, 1076–1082.

35. Pugazhendhi, A., Kumar, S.S., Manikandan, M., & Saravanan, M. Photocatalytic and antimicrobial efficacy of Fe doped CuO nanoparticles against the pathogenic bacteria and fungi. *Microbial Pathogenesis* (2018), 122, 84.

36. El Saeed, A.M., El-Fattah, M.A., Azzam, A.M., Dardir, M.M., & Bader, M.M. Synthesis of cuprous oxide epoxy nanocomposite as an environmentally antimicrobial coating. *International Journal of Biological Macromolecules* (2016), 89, 190–197.

37. Hsueh, Y.-H., Tsai, P.-H., & Lin, K.-S. pH-dependent antimicrobial properties of copper oxide nanoparticles in Staphylococcus aureus. *International Journal of Molecular Sciences* (2017), 18(4), 793. https://doi.org/10.3390/ijms18040793.

38. Sui, Y., Fu, W., Yang, H., Zeng, Y., Zhang, Y., Zhao, Q., Li, Y., Zhou, X., Leng, Y., Li, M., & Zou, G. Low temperature synthesis of Cu_2O crystals: Shape evolution and growth mechanism. *Crystal Growth and Design* (2010), 10(1), 99–108.

39. Gilbertson, L.M., Albalghiti, E.M., Fishman, Z.S., Perreault, F., Corredor, C., Posner, J.D., Elimelech, M., Pfefferle, L.D., & Zimmerman, J.B. Shape-dependent surface reactivity and antimicrobial activity of nano-cupric oxide. *Environmental Science and Technology* (2016), 50(7), 3975–3984.

40. Pang, H., Gao, F., & Lu, Q. Morphology effect on antibacterial activity of cuprous oxide. *Chemical Communications* (2009), 9(9), 1076–1078.

41. Mishchenko, T., Mitroshina, E., Balalaeva, I., Krysko, O., Vedunova, M., & Krysko, D. An emerging role for nanomaterials in increasing immunogenicity of cancer cell death. *Biochimica et biophysica acta (BBA) – Reviews on cancer* (2019), 1871(1), 99–108. https://doi.org/10. 1016/j.bbcan.2018.11.004.

42. Houskova, V., Stengl, V., Bakardjieva, S., Murafa, N., Kalendova, A., & Oplustil, F. Zinc oxide prepared by homogeneous hydrolysis with thioacetamide, its destruction of warfare agents, and photocatalytic activity. *Journal of Physical Chemistry. Part A* (2007), 111(20), 4215–4221. https://doi.org/10.1021/jp070878d.

43. Dadi, R., Azouani, R., Traore, M., Mielcarek, C., & Kanaev, A. Antibacterial activity of ZnO and CuO nanoparticles against gram positive and gram negative strains. *Materials Science and Engineering C – Materials for Biological Applications* (2019), 104, 109968. https://doi.org/10.1016/j.msec.2019.109968.

44. Agarwal, H., & Shanmugam, V. A review on anti-inflammatory activity of green synthesized zinc oxide nanoparticle: Mechanism-based approach. *Bioorganic Chemistry* (2020), 94, 103423. https://doi.org/10.1016/j.bioorg.2019.103423.

45. Nagajyothi, P.C., Cha, S.J., Yang, I.J., Sreekanth, T.V., Kim, K.J., & Shin, H.M. Antioxidant and anti-inflammatory activities of zinc oxide nanoparticles synthesized using Polygala tenuifolia root extract. *Journal of Photochemistry and Photobiology, Part B: Biology* (2015), 146, 10–17. https://doi.org/10.1016/j.jphotobiol.2015.02.008.

46. Mishra, P.K., Mishra, H., Ekielski, A., Talegaonkar, S., & Vaidya, B. Zinc oxide nanoparticles: A promising nanomaterial for biomedical applications. *Drug Discovery Today* (2017), 22(12), 1825–1834. https://doi.org/10.1016/j.drudis.2017.08.006.

47. Umrani, R.D., & Paknikar, K.M. Zinc oxide nanoparticles show antidiabetic activity in streptozotocin-induced Type 1 and 2 diabetic rats. *Nanomedicine* (2014), 9(1), 89–104. https://doi.org/10.2217/nnm.12.205.

48. El-Gharbawy, R.M., Emara, A.M., & Abu-Risha, S.E. Zinc oxide nanoparticles and a standard antidiabetic drug restore the function and structure of beta cells in type-2 diabetes. *Biomedicine and Pharmacotherapy* (2016), 84, 810–820. https://doi.org/10.1016/j.biopha.2016.09.068.

49. Dizaj, S.M., Lotfipour, F., Barzegar-Jalali, M., Zarrintan, M.H., & Adibkia, K. Antimicrobial activity of the metals and metal oxide nanoparticles. *Materials Science and Engineering: Part C* (2014), 44, 278–284.

50. Jin, S.-E., & Jin, H.-E. Synthesis, characterization, and three-dimensional structure generation of zinc oxide-based nanomedicine for biomedical applications. *Pharmaceutics* (2019), 11(11), 575.

51. Ul Haq, A.N., Nadhman, A., Ullah, I., Mustafa, G., Yasinzai, M., & Khan, I. Synthesis approaches of zinc oxide nanoparticles: The dilemma of ecotoxicity. *Journal of Nanomaterials* (2017), 2017, 8510342.

52. Sánchez-López, E., Gomes, D., Esteruelas, G., Bonilla, L., Lopez-Machado, A.L., Galindo, R., Cano, A., Espina, M., Ettcheto, M., Camins, A., Silva, A.M., Durazzo, A., Santini, A., Garcia, M.L., Souto, E.B. Metal-based nanoparticles as antimicrobial agents: An overview. *Nanomaterials* (2020), 10(2), 292.

53. Tamimi, N., Mohammadi Nafchi, A., Hashemi-Moghaddam, H., & Baghaie, H. The effects of nano-zinc oxide morphology on functional and antibacterial properties of tapioca starch bionanocomposite. *Food Science and Nutrition* (2021), 9(8), 4497–4508. https://doi.org/10.1002/fsn3.2426.

54. Yang, T., Oliver, S., Chen, Y., Boyer, C., & Chandrawati, R. Tuning, crystallization and morphology of zinc oxide with polyvinylpyrrolidone: Formation mechanisms and antimicrobial activity. *Journal of Colloid and Interface Science* (2019). https://doi.org/10.1016/j.jcis.2019.03.051.

55. Saliani, M., Jalal, R., & Kafshadre Goharshadi, E. Effects of pH and temperature on anti-bacterial activity of zinc oxide nanofluid against E. coli O157:H7 and Staphylococcus aureus. *Jundishapur Journal of Microbiology* (2015), 8(2). https://doi.org/10.5812/jjm.17115.

56. Raghupathi, K.R., Koodali, R.T., & Manna, A.C. Size-dependent bacterial growth inhibition and mechanism of antibacterial activity of zinc oxide nanoparticles. *Langmuir* (2011), 27(7), 4020–4028. https://doi.org/10.1021/la104825u.

57. Shanavas, S., Duraimurugan, J., Suresh Kumar, G., Ramesh, R., Acevedo, R., Anbarasan, P., & Maadeswaran, P. Ecofriendly green synthesis of ZnO nanostructures using Artabotrys Hexapetalu and Bambusa vulgaris plant extract and investigation on their photocatalytic and antibacterial activity. *Materials Research Express* (2019). https://doi.org/10.1088/2053-1591/ab3efe.

58. Jin, S.-E., Jin, J.E., Hwang, W., & Hong, S.W. Photocatalytic antibacterial application of zinc oxide nanoparticles and self-assembled networks under dual UV irradiation for enhanced disinfection. *International Journal of Nanomedicine* (2019), 14, 1737–1751. https://doi.org/10.2147/ijn.s192277.

59. Bala, N., Saha, S., Chakraborty, M., Maiti, M., Das, S., Basu, R., & Nandy, P. Green synthesis of zinc oxide nanoparticles using Hibiscus subdariffa leaf extract: Effect of temperature on synthesis, anti-bacterial activity and anti-diabetic activity. *RSC Advances* (2015), 5(7), 4993–5003. https://doi.org/10.1039/c4ra12784f.

60. Singh, J., Juneja, S., Palsaniya, S., Manna, A.K., Soni, R.K., & Bhattacharya, J. Evidence of oxygen defects mediated enhanced photocatalytic and antibacterial performance of ZnO nanorods. *Colloids and Surfaces, Part B: Biointerfaces* (2019), 184, 110541. https://doi.org/10.1016/j.colsurfb.2019.11054.

61. Ahmed, F., Arshi, N., Jeong, Y.S., Anwar, M.S., Dwivedi, S., Alsharaeh, E., & Koo, B.H. Novel Biomimatic synthesis of ZnO nanorods using egg white (albumen) and their antibacterial studies. *Journal of Nanoscience and Nanotechnology* (2016), 16(6), 5959–5965. https://doi.org/10.1166/jnn.2016.12127.

62. Chandra, H., Patel, D., Kumari, P., Jangwan, J.S., & Yadav, S. Phyto-mediated synthesis of zinc oxide nanoparticles of Berberis aristata: Characterization, antioxidant activity and antibacterial activity with special reference to urinary tract pathogens. *Materials Science and Engineering: Part C* (2019). https://doi.org/10.1016/j.msec.2019.04.035.

63. Elkady, M.F., Shokry Hassan, H., Hafez, E.E., & Fouad, A. Construction of zinc oxide into different morphological structures to be utilized as antimicrobial agent against multidrug resistant bacteria. *Bioinorganic Chemistry and Applications* (2015), 2015, 1–20. https://doi.org/10.1155/2015/536854.

64. López de Dicastillo, C., Patiño Vidal, C., Falcó, I., Sánchez, G., Márquez, P., & Escrig, J. Antimicrobial bilayer nanocomposites based on the incorporation of as-synthetized hollow zinc oxide nanotubes. *Nanomaterials* (2020), 10(3), 503. https://doi.org/10.3390/nano10030503.

65. Cavassin, E.D., de Figueiredo, L.F.P., Otoch, J.P., Seckler, M.M., de Oliveira, R.A., Franco, F.F., Marangoni, V.S., Zucolotto, V., Levin, A.S.S., & Costa, S.F. Comparison of methods to detect the in vitro activity of silver nanoparticles (AgNP) against multidrug resistant bacteria. *Journal of Nanobiotechnology* (2015), 13, 1–16.

66. Silva, L.P., Silveira, A.P., Bonatto, C.C., Reis, I.G., & Milreu, P.V. Silver nanoparticles as antimicrobial agents: Past, present, and future. In: *Nanostructures for Antimicrobial Therapy: Nanostructures in Therapeutic Medicine Series*; Ficai, Anton, Grumezescu, Alexandru, Ed.; Amsterdam: Elsevier, pp. 577–596, 2017. ISBN: 9780323461511.

67. Tong, J.W. Case reports on the use of antimicrobial (silver impregnated) soft silicone foam dressing on infected diabetic foot ulcers. *International Wound Journal* (2009), 6(4), 275–284.

68. Miller, C.N., Newall, N., Kapp, S.E., Lewin, G., Karimi, L., Carville, K., Gliddon, T., & Santamaria, N.M. A randomized-controlled trial comparing cadexomer iodine and nanocrystalline silver on the healing of leg ulcers. *Wound Repair and Regeneration* (2010), 18(4), 359–367.

69. Castellano, J.J., Shafii, S.M., Ko, F., Donate, G., Wright, T.E., Mannari, R.J., Payne, W.G., Smith, D.J., & Robson, M.C. Comparative evaluation of silver-containing antimicrobial dressings and drugs. *International Wound Journal* (2007), 4(2), 114–122.

70. Kim, Y.T., Kim, K., Han, J.H., & Kimmel, R.M. Antimicrobial active packaging for food. In: *Smart Packaging Technologies for Fast Moving Consumer Goods* (2008), 76, 99–110. doi.org/10.1002/9780470753699.ch6

71. Kampmann, Y., De Clerck, E., Kohn, S., Patchala, D.K., Langerock, R., & Kreyenschmidt, J. Study on the antimicrobial effect of silver-containing inner liners in refrigerators. *Journal of Applied Microbiology* (2008), 104(6), 1808–1814.

72. Kędziora, A., Speruda, M., Krzyzewska, E., Rybka, J., Łukowiak, A., & Bugla-Płoskońska, G. Similarities and differences between silver ions and silver in nanoforms as antibacterial agents. *International Journal of Molecular Sciences* (2018), 19, 444.

73. Yaqoob, A.A., Ahmad, H., Parveen, T., Ahmad, A., Oves, M., Ismail, I.M.I., Qari, H.A., Umar, K., & Mohamad Ibrahim, M.N. Recent advances in metal decorated nanomaterials and their various biological applications: A review. *Frontiers in Chemistry* (2020), 8, 341.

74. Kulkarni, S.K. *Nanotechnology—Principles and Practices*, 3rd ed.; Berlin: Springer, 2014. ISBN 9783319091709.

75. Tran, Q.H., Nguyen, V.Q., & Le, A. Silver nanoparticles: Synthesis, properties, toxicology, applications and perspectives. *Advances in Natural Sciences: Nanoscience and Nanotechnology* (2013), 4(3), 033001.

76. Argueta Figueroa, L., Arenas-Arrocena, M.C., Díaz–Herrera, A.P., García-Benítez, S.V., & García-Contreras, R. Propiedades antimicrobianas y citotóxicas de un adhesivo de uso ortodóncico adicionado con nanopartículas de plata. *Mundo nano. Revista interdisciplinaria en nanociencias y nanotecnología* (2018), 12(22), 1.

77. Marambio-Jones, C., & Hoek, E.M.V. A review of the antibacterial effects of silver nanomaterials and potential implications for human health and the environment. *Journal of Nanoparticle Research* (2010), 12(5), 1531–1551.

78. Qing, Y., Cheng, L., Li, R., Liu, G., Zhang, Y., Tang, X., Wang, J., Liu, H., & Qin, Y. Potential antibacterial mechanism of silver nanoparticles and the optimization of orthopedic implants by advanced modification technologies. *International Journal of Nanomedicine* (2018), 13, 3311–3327.

79. Dakal, T.C., Kumar, A., Majumdar, R.S., & Yadav, V. Mechanistic basis of antimicrobial actions of silver nanoparticles. *Frontiers in Microbiology* (2016), 7, 1831.
80. Seong, M., & Lee, D.G. Silver nanoparticles against Salmonella enterica serotype Typhimurium: Role of inner membrane dysfunction. *Current Microbiology* (2017), 74(6), 661–670.
81. Ivask, A., Elbadawy, A., Kaweeteerawat, C., Boren, D., Fischer, H., Ji, Z., Chang, C.H., Liu, R., Tolaymat, T., Telesca, D., Zink, J.I., Cohen, Y., Holden, P.A., & Godwin, H.A. Toxicity mechanisms in Escherichia coli vary for silver nanoparticles and differ from ionic silver. *ACS Nano* (2014), 8(1), 374–386.
82. Seil, J.T., & Webster, T.J. Antimicrobial applications of nanotechnology: Methods and literature. *International Journal of Nanomedicine* (2012), 7, 2767–2781.
83. Crisan, C.M., Mocan, T., Manolea, M., Lasca, L.I., Tăbăran, F.-A., & Mocan, L. Review on silver nanoparticles as a novel class of antibacterial solutions. *Applied Sciences* (2021), 11(3), 1120. https://doi.org/10.3390/app11031120.
84. Tang, S., & Zheng, J. Antibacterial activity of silver nanoparticles: Structural effects. *Advanced Healthcare Materials* (2018), 7(13), 1701503.
85. Roelofs, D., Makama, S., De Boer, T.E., Vooijs, R., Van Gestel, C.A., & Van Den Brink, N.W. Surface coating and particle size are main factors explaining the transcriptome-wide responses of the earthworm Lumbricus rubellus to silver nanoparticles. *Environmental Science: Nano* (2020), 7(4), 1179–1193.
86. Casey, B.J., & Dair, B.J. Influence of size on antimicrobial activity of silver nanoparticles. *Advanced Science, Engineering and Medicine* (2015), 7(2), 112–119.
87. Dong, Y., Zhu, H., Shen, Y., Zhang, W., & Zhang, L. Antibacterial activity of silver nanoparticles of different particle size against Vibrio natriegens. *PLOS ONE* (2019), 14(9), e0222322. https://doi.org/10.1371/journal.pone.0222322.
88. Tang, S., Meng, X., Lu, H., & Zhu, S. PVP-assisted sonoelectrochemical growth of silver nanostructures with various shapes. *Materials Chemistry and Physics* (2009), 116(2–3), 464–468. https://doi.org/10.1016/j.matchemphys.2009.04.
89. Gao, M., Sun, L., Wang, Z., & Zhao, Y. Controlled synthesis of Ag nanoparticles with different morphologies and their antibacterial properties. *Materials Science and Engineering: Part C* (2013), 33(1), 397–404. https://doi.org/10.1016/j.msec.2012.09.005.
90. Slepička, P., Slepičková Kasálková, N., Siegel, J., Kolská, Z., & Švorčík, V. Methods of gold and silver nanoparticles preparation. *Materials* (2019), 13(1), 1. https://doi.org/10.3390/ma13010001.
91. Osonga, F.J., Akgul, A., Yazgan, I., Akgul, A., Eshun, G.B., Sakhaee, L., & Sadik, O.A. Size and shape-dependent antimicrobial activities of silver and gold nanoparticles: A model study as potential fungicides. *Molecules* (2020), 25(11), 2682. https://doi.org/10.3390/molecules25112682.
92. Zhu, S., Shen, Y., Yu, Y., & Bai, X. Synthesis of antibacterial gold nanoparticles with different particle sizes using chlorogenic acid. *Royal Society Open Science* (2020), 7(3), 191141. https://doi.org/10.1098/rsos.191141.
93. Penders, J., Stolzoff, M., Hickey, D.J., Andersson, M., & Webster, T.J. Shape-dependent antibacterial effects of non-cytotoxic gold nanoparticles. *International Journal of Nanomedicine* (2017), 12, 2457–2468. https://doi.org/10.2147/ijn.s124442.
94. Hameed, S., Wang, Y., Zhao, L., Xie, L., & Ying, Y. Shape-dependent significant physical mutilation and antibacterial mechanisms of gold nanoparticles against foodborne bacterial pathogens (Escherichia coli, Pseudomonas aeruginosa and Staphylococcus aureus) at lower concentrations. *Materials Science and Engineering: Part C* (2020), 108, 110338. https://doi.org/10.1016/j.msec.2019.110338.

3 Antiviral Polymers For Food Safety

Ruby Varghese, Namitha Vijay,
and Yogesh Bharat Dalvi

CONTENTS

3.1 INTRODUCTION

Phenomenological craving for food has grown nearly to 100% in young women and 70% in men in recent years (Weingarten, and Elston, 1991, Splane et al., 2019). Along with this phenomenon, a series of syndromes have been highlighted, where food poisoning steals the limelight.

This has paved the way for the onset of many gastroenteric diseases and hepatitis bringing human enteroviruses such as human norovirus (HuNoroVs), astroviruses, rotavirus, and sapoviruses to scientific attention (Randazzo et al., 2018). These viruses not only cause gastroenteritis but also cause additional disorders such as Hepatitis A Virus (HAV), hepatitis E virus (HEV), poliomyelitis, and meningitis which eventually leads to the morbidity and mortality of impuissant populations such as children, immunocompromised patients, pregnant women, and aged individuals (Rodriguez et al., 2012). However, food poisoning caused by viruses has received lesser attention than other foodborne pathogens such as *Campylobacter*, *Clostridium perfringens*, *Escherichia coli*, *Listeria*, and *Salmonella*. Over the years

DOI: 10.1201/9781003243175-3

from a food perspective, viruses have emerged as an infectious agent which causes approximately 600 million cases of illness annually (WHO, 2015).

One of the important modes of transmission of the pathogen is the contamination caused by food packaging. This eventually led to research on food-grade polymers as edible outer covering and packaging material (Bianculli et al., 2020).

Microbiological food safety and quality can be improved by the incorporation of antimicrobial or antiviral agents into these food-grade polymers (Carbone et al., 2016). Recently researchers have spotted the importance of food-grade additives developed from natural polymers. Natural extracts such as green tea extract (GTE) (Amankwaah et al., 2020 a), grape seed extract (GSE) (Amankwaah et al., 2020b), essential oils (Efrati et al. 2014 and Maurya et al., 2021), and polyphenols (Zhu, 2021) are excellent candidates for the development of food-grade polymers. These additives not only keep the food from getting spoiled but also exhibit antioxidant, antimicrobial, and antiviral properties.

Natural polymers for packaging include proteins, lipids, and a variety of polysaccharides which can increase the shelf life of the food products. These biomolecules can be tailored and customized accordingly to combat various bacteria, pathogen fungi, and mostly enteric viruses (Randazzo et al., 2018).

The development of food-grade polymers with antiviral activity for food applications will be a topic of interest for both academia and the food industry to enhance microbial safety. The present review compiles published literature in this widely unexplored area and highlights the current state of knowledge.

3.2   MOST IMPORTANT FOODBORNE VIRUSES

Viruses do not produce toxins or do not multiply in food like other microorganisms. Food acts as a vehicle for the transmission of viruses. Major contributors of viral borne food diseases are Hepatitis A Virus (HAV) and Human Norovirus (NoV) while others include enterovirus, human rotavirus, Hepatitis E Virus (HEV), astrovirus, Aichi Virus (AiV) Sapovirus, coronavirus, parvovirus, and human adenovirus (HAdV) (Petrović and D'Agostino, 2016 and EFSA, 2011). These viruses are small, and contain single-stranded (+) ve sense RNA or DNA virus or ds RNA without a lipid envelope. Details of some of the viruses transmitted through food are enlisted below:

3.2.1   HUMAN NOROVIRUS (NoV)

A major contributor to foodborne disease which causes epidemic gastroenteritis. The virus is mainly observed in the stools and vomit of infected people, and is transmitted through person-person interaction. Food like oysters and imported raspberries are vehicles of NoV transmission (Petrović, 2013).

3.2.2   HEPATITIS A VIRUS (HAV)

One of the major contributors to foodborne diseases. HAV is transmitted from person to person by those engaged in sexual activity, who have consumed contaminated food, or are exposed to, or maintain, insufficient hygiene. It may also be transmitted from food handlers or food processors (Bosch, 1998; Pebody et al., 1998; Lees, 2000; Greening, 2006; Cook and Rzeźutka, 2006; Tallon et al., 2008; Petrović et al., 2013, 2016). HAV has a prolonged incubation period of two to six weeks, thus before symptoms become apparent HAV is shed. Foodborne outbreaks via HAV are not so prevalent in developing countries as they acquire herd immunity as compared to people in developed countries who are not vaccinated (Greening, 2006).

3.2.3 HEPATITIS E VIRUS (HEV)

This is most commonly observed in the Indian subcontinent, China, and Central Asia. It is susceptible to spread zoonotically in industrial countries (Bosch et al., 2008). The main route of HEV transmission is a faecal-oral route, mostly via the consumption of water contaminated with faeces (Greening, 2006; FAO/WHO, 2008).

3.2.4 HUMAN ROTAVIRUS VIRUS (HRV)

Highly prevalent in most countries and which accounts for more than 130 million cases of diarrhoea in children (<5) annually (Glass and Kilgore, 1997). It mostly occurs during winter or colder conditions and drier months. HRV is transmitted through the consumption of contaminated water and food or contact with contaminated surfaces as HRV is stable in the environment (Greening, 2006).

3.2.5 HUMAN ENTERIC VIRUS

Poliovirus is one such enteric virus which was reported to be the first foodborne pathogen (Jubb, 1915; Sattar and Tetro, 2001). However, presently foodborne transmission via the poliovirus is not seen due to the absence of virulent wild-type pathogens.

3.2.6 ASTROVIRUS

This is prevalent in both animals and humans. It is transmitted via contaminated water or food and from an infected person to a healthy person. It causes self-limiting gastroenteritis for both humans and animals (Appleton, 2001).

3.3 POLYMER AND BIOPOLYMERS AS ACTIVE CARRIERS OF ANTIMICROBIAL/ANTIVIRAL COMPOUNDS

Food polymers are designed to enhance the technological advancements of packaging materials to improve food safety and extend the shelf life of food products. The mode of action of these polymers is by inhibiting growth and the multiplication of microorganisms as well as restricting the spoilage of food products. The encapsulation of active compounds within the polymer or the binding of therapeutic agents to the polymer through covalent bonding will ensure its efficacy (Su et al., 2015).

Various factors need to be considered while designing antiviral polymers. Some of them are briefed below:

1. Type of material to be used.
2. Chemical composition, polarity, and molecular weight of polymers.
3. Processing conditions for the designing of materials nowhere should affect the overall efficacy of antiviral compounds.
4. Type of interaction with the bounded active compounds.
5. The polymeric material should be non-toxic, preferably biodegradable, and biocompatible as well as not interfere with the release of antimicrobial (antiviral) compounds.

3.4   ANTIMICROBIAL FOOD PACKAGING

The transference of a virus through food is quite easy, as the mode of transmission could be during processing, transportation, and ultimately during consumption. Various viruses like the coronavirus and the human rotavirus remain on surfaces for several days (Mallakpour et al., 2021).

Martíinez-Abad and collaborators (Martíinez-Abad et al., 2013) were the first group of researchers to develop a polylactic acid (PLA) incorporating silver ions-based food-packaging material which exhibited against the surrogate strain feline calicivirus (FCV).

The incorporation of metals with food-grade polymeric materials has significant potential applications. Bright et al., 2008, impregnated plastic coupons with zeolite powder containing copper and silver metals which exhibited an antiviral effect against FCV.

With the advancement of nanotechnology, some researchers included nanoparticles with a food-grade polymeric material to explore its potential. Park et al., 2014 fabricated a novel micrometer-sized magnetic hybrid colloid (MHC) that displayed antiviral effects against bacteriophage, MNV, and adenovirus. Meanwhile, in another study Castro-Mayogra et al., 2017, developed poly (3-hydroxybutyrate-CO-3 hydroxy valerate) with silver nanoparticles which displayed a virucidal effect against HuNoV, FCV, and MNV. In another study, Dominguez et al., 2020 developed photocatalytic coatings with HCl and Titanium oxide nanoparticles which impart antimicrobial properties. This fabricated coating eventually prevents spoilage and cross-contamination.

Several researchers like Noyce et al., 2007; Manuel et al., 2015, Borkow and Gabbay, 2004; Ditta et al., 2008 and Castro-Mayogra et al., 2017 have shown the antiviral effect of copper alone or copper incorporated synthetic polymers against HuNoV, HIV-1, Bacteriophage-T4, and MNV.

In a recent study, a novel continuously active antimicrobial coating displayed a virucidal effect against the human coronavirus (HCoV) 229E (Ikner et al., 2020).

Mizielińska et al., 2021 fabricated polyethylene covering made up of ZnO nanoparticles containing geraniol or carvacrol which showed moderate virucidal effects against the phi 6 phage (used as a surrogate for viruses) by extending the food quality and freshness of food products.

Various other researchers also investigated the virus inhibitory activity of zinc metal against surrogate strains such as HIV-1 (Haraguchi et al., 1999); HSV (Arens and Travis, 2000), rhinovirus (Hulisz, 2004), respiratory syncytial virus (Suara and Crowe, 2004), and MNV (Warnes and Keevil, 2013).

Polyaniline and polypyrrole are conducting polymers which are excellent food coating materials due to their microbial resistance properties (Balasubramaniam et al., 2020). Synthetic and bio-based plastics like propylene or polyhydroxyalkanoates are used as food packaging material. Pyridinium-type polyvinylpyrrolidones showed antiviral activity against the influenza virus with a virucidal efficiency of 95.6% (Xue and Xiao, 2015).

3.5　EDIBLE POLYMERS

Edible polymers are derived from natural sources which are conventionally considered waste or discarded materials. Some of the edible polymers are enlisted in Table 3.1. The advantages of edible polymer over synthetic polymer are: (a) commonly available/ abundant in the biosphere, (b) low-cost, (c) biodegradable and recyclable, (d) thermo processable (Salleh et al., 2009), (e) provides a good barrier to moisture, oxygen, and the movement of solutes for the food (Mokrejs et al., 2009), (f) non-toxic, and (g) reduce environmental contamination.

Certain edible biopolymers such as Zein and soy protein; beeswax, chitosan, starch, and cellulose which are protein, lipid, and carbohydrates are preferred for food packaging material as they fulfill the criteria of GRAS (generally recognized as safe) status.

Some of the postulated candidates with potential antiviral effects are natural extracts such as green tea extract (GTE), grape seed extract (GSE), and secondary metabolites such as curcumin, polyphenol etc. (Li et al., 2013; D'Souza, 2014; Ryu et al., 2015)

Chen et al., 2020 added curcumin into the polyvinyl acetate matrix which imparts antimicrobial activity against *Salmonella typhimurium* and *S. aureus* while another study by Li et al., 2020 demonstrated that Carboxymethyl cellulose/montmorillonite clay/ε-poly-(L-lysine) nanocomposite films displayed antimicrobial activity against fungi (*Botrytis cinerea* and *Rhizopus oligosporus*) and bacteria (*S. aureus, and E. Coli*). These compounds which showed antimicrobial activities have the definite potential to inhibit viral growth days (Mallakpour et al., 2021).

Amankwaah et al., 2020 developed chitosan-based food packaging material containing grape seed extract (GSE). This fabricated coating imparted antiviral activity by inhibiting or restricting the growth or replication of Murine NoroVirus-1 (MNV-1). Additionally, this packaging material also exhibited antibacterial activity against *Escherichia coli* and *Listeria innocua*.

TABLE 3.1

Edible Polymers and Their Properties

S. No.	Edible biopolymer	Source	Properties	Application in food industry
1.	Hydrocolloid			
A.	Starch	Cereal grain and tuber	Odourless, tasteless, colourless, non-toxic, biologically absorbable, semipermeable to CO_2 and resistance to oxygen	Food packaging (Utami et al., 2014)
B.	Alginate	Seaweed	Unique colloidal property (Rhim, 2004)	Used as a thickener in food like soup and jellies
C.	Carrageenans	Red seaweed	Increased viscosity	Used in desserts, sauces, beer, toothbrushes etc.
D.	Carboxymethyl cellulose	Cellulose-derivative	Flexible, tasteless, colourless, water-soluble, moderate barrier to O_2	Biodegradable packaging material (Wang et al., 2000 and Coma et al., 2003)
E.	Chitosan	Exoskeleton of crustaceans	Biodegradable, chemically inert, high mechanical strength, low cost (Mucha et al., 2007 and)	Biodegradable packaging material
2.	Polypeptide			
A.	Gelatin	Animal	High content of amino acids like glycine, proline, and hydroxy proline Hydrophilic in nature Reduces O_2, moisture, and transport of oil	Biodegradable packaging material Coatings on meat (Khan et al., 2013)
B.	Zein	Plant	Reduce moisture and loss of firmness	Biodegradable packaging material – delay colour alterations in fresh fruits. Also used as crust in candy, nuts, fruits etc. (Dhanya et al., 2012)
2.	Lipids			
A.	Shellac resins	Secretion of *Lacciferlacca*	Reduce O_2, moisture	Food packaging (Bourtroom, 2008)
B.	Rosin	Plant	Reduce moisture and keep fruits fresh	Coating on citrus fruits (Berg et al., 2012)

3.6 ASSAYS TO EVALUATE THE ANTIVIRAL ACTIVITY OF FOOD POLYMERS

The virucidal effect can be evaluated by adding a known amount of a virus to a given polymeric material followed by assessing the reduction in virus titer, and determining the significance of viral decay using standard statistical procedures (Randazzo et al., 2018).

The in vitro cultivation of human enteric viruses such as HuNoV or a wild-type HAV strain is a difficult task, hence for viral detection surrogate strains such as the feline calicivirus (FCV), MNV, and Tulane Virus (TNV) (Hirneisen and Kniel, 2013) are used. The most limiting objective in using surrogate strains is the validity of these strains as models, hence the need for them to be carefully assessed (Bae and Schwab, 2008; NACMCF, 2016)

Virus detection is carried out through cell culture by implementing various assays such as:

1. Formation of cytopathic effects.
2. Plaque assays.
3. Tissue culture infectious dose 50 ($TCID_{50}$).

The standard procedure employed to evaluate the virucidal effect of polymeric food packaging material is as follows:

1. Apply or add viral inoculation onto the material.
2. Incubation time for exerting antiviral activity by the material.
3. Addition of neutralization solution to stop the inhibition action (Bright et al., 2009; Martínez-Abad et al., 2013).
4. Finally, compare the test material with a control (polymeric material without antiviral coating).

This procedure cannot be employed for coatings as its gel nature may complicate the assessment process, hence for the coatings following steps are required:

1. Incubation of coating with viral suspension (diluted in PBS) overnight at 37°C.
2. Addition of neutralization solution to stop the inhibition action (Bright et al., 2009; Martínez-Abad et al., 2013).
3. Finally, viruses were titrated in the corresponding cell line (Randazzo et al., 2018).

There are many parameters to be considered to develop methodologies for the assessment of antiviral properties and they are as follows:

1. Type and characteristic property of the active (antiviral) compound.
2. Type of binding of the active (antiviral) compound with a polymeric material.

3. Evaluation of toxicity of polymeric material using cell lines.
4. Assessment of viral contact time with a polymeric material.
5. Effect of neutralization solution.
6. Determination of experimental conditions used like temperature, humidity etc.
7. Techniques adapted for viral recovery.

3.7 CONCLUSION

Foodborne viral contamination is a serious health and economic problem. Currently, the viral inactivation process employed does not only inhibit viruses but may also affect the quality of food. Hence, the following measures need to be taken for an effective reduction in diseases associated with the enteric virus through food:

1. Advanced food processing strategies.
2. Innovative sanitation procedures/approaches.
3. Consumer awareness.

Hence, the development of biopolymers with antiviral activity for food packaging is an open field of research that needs to be fully addressed.

REFERENCES

Amankwaah, C., Li, J., Lee, J., & Pascall, M. A. (2020a). Antimicrobial activity of chitosan-based films enriched with green tea extracts on murine Norovirus, Escherichia coli, and Listeria innocua. *International Journal of Food Science*, 2020 Article ID 3941924,1-9.

Amankwaah, C., Li, J., Lee, J., & Pascall, M. A. (2020b). Development of antiviral and bacteriostatic chitosan-based food packaging material with grape seed extract for murine Norovirus, Escherichia coli, and Listeria innocua control. *Food Science and Nutrition*, 8(11), 6174–6181.

Appleton, H. (2001). Norwalk virus and the small round viruses causing food-borne gastroenteritis. In: Hui, Y. H., Sattar, S. A., Murrell, K. D., Nip, W. K., & Stanfield, P. S. (Eds.), *Food-borne Disease Handbook: Viruses, Parasites, Pathogens and HACCP*, 2nd ed., vol. 2. Marcel Dekker, New York, pp. 77–97.

Arens, M., & Travis, S. (2000). Zinc salts inactivate clinical isolates of herpes simplex virus in vitro. *Journal of Clinical Microbiology*, 38(5), 1758–1762.

Bae, J., & Schwab, K. J. (2008). Evaluation of murine Norovirus, feline calicivirus, poliovirus, and MS2 as surrogates for human Norovirus in a model of viral persistence in surface water and groundwater. *Applied and Environmental Microbiology*, 74(2), 477–484.

Balasubramaniam, B., Prateek, Ranjan, S., Saraf, M., Kar, P., Singh, S. P., Thakur, V. K., Singh, A., & Gupta, R. K. (2020). Antibacterial and antiviral functional materials: Chemistry and biological activity toward tackling COVID-19-like pandemics. *ACS Pharmacology & Translational Science*, 4(1), 8–54.

Berg, S., Bretz, M., Hubbermann, E. M., & Schwarz, K. (2012). Influence of different pectins on powder characteristics of microencapsulated anthocyanins and their impact on drug retention of shellac coated granulate. *Journal of Food Engineering*, 108(1), 158–165.

Bianculli, R. H., Mase, J. D., & Schulz, M. D. (2020). Antiviral polymers: Past approaches and future possibilities. *Macromolecules*, 53(21), 9158–9186.

Bianculli, R. H., Mase, J. D., & Schulz, M. D. (2020). Antiviral polymers: Past approaches and future possibilities. *Macromolecules*, 53(21), 9158–9186.

Biology and Food Safety, vol. XVIII. Springer, New York, pp. 5–42.

Borkow, G., & Gabbay, J. (2004). Putting copper into action: Copper-impregnated products with potent biocidal activities. *The FASEB Journal*, 18(14), 1728–1730.

Bosch, A. (1998). Human enteric viruses in the water environment: A minireview. *International Microbiology*, 1(3), 191–196.

Bosch, A., Guix, S., Sano, D., & Pinto, R. M. (2008). New tools for the study and direct surveillance of viral pathogens in water. *Current Opinion in Biotechnology*, 19(3), 295–301.

Bourtoom, T. (2008). Edible films and coatings: Characteristics and properties. *International Food Research Journal*, 15(3), 237–248.

Bright, K. R., Sicairos-Ruelas, E. E., Gundy, P. M., & Gerba, C. P. (2009). Assessment of the antiviral properties of zeolites containing metal ions. *Food and Environmental Virology*, 1(1), 37–41.

Carbone, M., Donia, D. T., Sabbatella, G., & Antiochia, R. (2016, October 1). Silver nanoparticles in polymeric matrices for fresh food packaging. *Journal of King Saud University – Science*, 28(4), 273–279.

Castro-Mayorga, J. L., Randazzo, W., Fabra, M. J., Lagaron, J. M., Aznar, R., & Sánchez, G. (2017). Antiviral properties of silver nanoparticles against Norovirus surrogates and their efficacy in coated polyhydroxyalkanoates systems. *LWT – Food Science and Technology*, 79, 503–510.

Chen, L., Song, Z., Zhi, X., & Du, B. (2020). Photoinduced antimicrobial activity of curcumin-containing coatings: Molecular interaction, stability and potential application in food decontamination. *ACS Omega*, 5(48), 31044–31054.

Coma, V., Sebti, I., Pardon, P., Pichavant, F. H., & Deschamps, A. (2003, February 15). Deschamps A. Film properties from crosslinking of cellulosic derivatives with a polyfunctional carboxylic acid. *Carbohydrate Polymers*, 51(3), 265–271.

Cook, N., & Rzeźutka, A. (2006). Hepatitis viruses. In: Motarjemi, Y. & Adams, M. (Eds.), *Emerging Food-borne Pathogens*. Woodhead Publishing Limited, Cambridge, pp. 282–308.

Dhanya, A. T., Haridas, K. R., Divia, N., & Sudheesh, S. (2012). Development of Zein-Pectin nanoparticle as drug carrier. *International Journal of Drug Delivery*, 4(2), 147.

Ditta, I. B., Steele, A., Liptrot, C., Tobin, J., Tyler, H., Yates, H. M., Sheel, D. W., & Foster, H. A. (2008). Photocatalytic antimicrobial activity of thin surface films of TiO_2, CuO and TiO_2/CuO dual layers on Escherichia coli and bacteriophage T4. *Applied Microbiology and Biotechnology*, 79(1), 127–133.

Dominguez, E. T., Nguyen, P., Hylen, A., Maschmann, M. R., Mustapha, A., & Hunt, H. K. (2020). Design and characterization of mechanically stable, nanoporous TiO_2 thin film antimicrobial coatings for food contact surfaces. *Materials Chemistry and Physics*, 251, 123001.

D'Souza, D. H. (2014). Phytocompounds for the control of human enteric viruses. *Current Opinion in Virology*, 4, 44–49.

Efrati, R., Natan, M., Pelah, A., Haberer, A., Banin, E., Dotan, A., & Ophir, A. (2014). The effect of polyethylene crystallinity and polarity on thermal stability and controlled release of essential oils in antimicrobial films. *Journal of Applied Polymer Science*, 131(11), 1–11.

EFSA, Panel on Biological Hazards. (2011). Scientific opinion on an update on the present knowledge on the occurrence and control of foodborne viruses. *EFSA Journal*, 9,2190–2286.

FAO/WHO. (2008). Viruses in food: Scientific advice to support risk management activities. Meeting report microbiological risk assessment series, No. 13.

Glass, R. I., & Kilgore, P. E. (1997). Etiology of acute viral gastroenteritis. In: Gracey, M. & Walker-Smith, J. A. (Eds.), *Diarrheal Disease*, vol. 38. Vevey/Lippincott-Raven, Philadelphia, PA, pp. 39–53.

Greening, G. E. (2006). Human and animal viruses in food (including taxonomy of enteric viruses). In: Sagar, G. (Ed.), *Viruses in Foods*, Springer, Cham, pp. 5–57.

Haraguchi, Y., Sakurai, H., Hussain, S., Anner, B. M., & Hoshino, H. (1999). Inhibition of HIV-1 infection by zinc group metal compounds. *Antiviral Research*, 43(2), 123–133.

Hirneisen, K. A., & Kniel, K. E. (2013). Comparing human Norovirus surrogates: Murine Norovirus and Tulane virus. *Journal of Food Protection*, 76(1), 139–143.

Hulisz, D. (2004). Efficacy of zinc against common cold viruses: An overview. *Journal of the American Pharmacists Association*, 44(5), 594–603.

Ikner, L. A., Torrey, J. R., Gundy, P. M., & Gerba, C. P. (2020). *A Continuously Active Antimicrobial Coating Effective against Human Coronavirus 229E*, 20097329, 1–9. medRxiv.

Jubb, G. (1915). A third outbreak of epidemic poliomyelitis at West Kirby. *Lancet*, 185(4767), 67.

Khan, M. I., Adrees, M. N., Tariq, M. R., & Muhammad, S. (2013). Application of edible coating for improving meat quality: A review. *Pakistan Journal of Food Sciences*, 23(2), 71–79.

Lees, D. (2000). Viruses and bivalve shellfish. *International Journal of Food Microbiology*, 59(1–2), 81–116.

Li, D., Baert, L., & Uyttendaele, M. (2013). Inactivation of food-borne viruses using natural biochemical substances. *Food Microbiology*, 35(1), 1–9.

Mallakpour, S., Azadi, E., & Hussain, C. M. (2021). Recent breakthroughs of antibacterial and antiviral protective polymeric materials during COVID-19 pandemic and post-pandemic: Coating, packaging, and textile applications. *Current Opinion in Colloid and Interface Science*, 55, 101480.

Manuel, C. S., Moore, M. D., & Jaykus, L. A. (2015). Destruction of the capsid and genome of GII. 4 Human Norovirus occurs during exposure to metal alloys containing copper. *Applied and Environmental Microbiology*, 81(15), 4940–4946.

Martínez-Abad, A., Ocio, M. J., Lagarón, J. M., & Sánchez, G. (2013, March 1). Evaluation of silver-infused polylactide films for inactivation of Salmonella and feline calicivirus in vitro and on fresh-cut vegetables. *International Journal of Food Microbiology*, 162(1), 89–94.

Maurya, A., Prasad, J., Das, S., & Dwivedy, A. K. (2021). Essential oils and their application in food safety. *Frontiers in Sustainable Food Systems*, 5, 133.

Mizielińska, M., Nawrotek, P., Stachurska, X., Ordon, M., & Bartkowiak, A. (2021). Packaging covered with antiviral and antibacterial coatings based on ZnO nanoparticles supplemented with geraniol and carvacrol. *International Journal of Molecular Sciences*, 22(4), 1717.

Mokrejs, P., Langmaier, F., Janacova, D., Mladek, M., Kolomaznik, K., & Vasek, V. (2009). Thermal study and solubility tests of films based on amaranth flour starch–protein hydrolysate. *Journal of Thermal Analysis and Calorimetry*, 98(1), 299–307.

Mucha, M., Wańkowicz, K., & Balcerzak, J. (2007). Analysis of water adsorption on chitosan and its blends with hydroxypropylcellulose. *e-Polymers*, 7(1), 1–10.

National Advisory Committee on Microbiological Criteria for Foods. (2016). Response to the questions posed by the food safety and inspection service, the centers for disease control and prevention, the national marine fisheries service, and the defense health agency, veterinary services activity regarding control strategies for reducing foodborne norovirus infections. *Journal of Food Protection*, 79(5), 843–889.

Noyce, J. O., Michels, H., & Keevil, C. W. (2007). Inactivation of influenza A virus on copper versus stainless steel surfaces. *Applied and Environmental Microbiology*, 73(8), 2748–2750.

Park, S., Park, H. H., Kim, S. Y., Kim, S. J., Woo, K., & Ko, G. (2014). Antiviral properties of silver nanoparticles on a magnetic hybrid colloid. *Applied and Environmental Microbiology*, 80(8), 2343–2350.

Pebody, R. G., Leino, T., Ruutu, P., Kinnunen, L., Davidkin, I., Nohynek, H., & Leinikki, P. (1998). Food-borne outbreaks of hepatitis A in a low endemic country: An emerging problem? *Epidemiology and Infection*, 120(1), 55–59.

Petrović, T. (2013). Prevalence of viruses in food and the environment. In: Cook, N. (Ed.), *Viruses in Food and Water: Risks, Surveillance and Control*. Woodhead Publishing Limited, London, pp. 19–46.

Petrović, T., & D'Agostino, M. (2016). Viral contamination of food. In: *Antimicrobial Food Packaging*; Barros-Velázquez J., Ed.; Spain: Academic Press, pp. 65–79.

Randazzo, W., Fabra, M. J., Falcó, I., López-Rubio, A., & Sánchez, G. (2018). Polymers and biopolymers with antiviral activity: Potential applications for improving food safety. *Comprehensive Reviews in Food Science and Food Safety*, 17(3), 754–768.

Rhim, J. W. (2004). Physical and mechanical properties of water resistant sodium alginate films. *LWT – Food Science and Technology*, 37(3), 323–330.

Rodriguez-Lazaro, D., Cook, N., Ruggeri, F. M., Sellwood, J., Nasser, A., Nascimento, M. S., D'Agostino, M., Santos, R., Saiz, J. C., Rzeżutka, A., Bosch, A., Gironés, R., Carducci, A., Muscillo, M., Kovač, K., Diez-Valcarce, M., Vantarakis, A., von Bonsdorff, C. H., de Roda Husman, A. M., Hernández, M., & van der Poel, W. H. (2012). Virus hazards from food, water and other contaminated environments. *FEMS Microbiology Reviews*, 36(4), 786–814.

Ryu, S., You, H. J., Kim, Y. W., Lee, A., Ko, G. P., Lee, S. J., & Song, M. J. (2015). Inactivation of Norovirus and surrogates by natural phytochemicals and bioactive substances. *Molecular Nutrition and Food Research*, 59(1), 65–74.

Salleh, E., Muhamad, I. I., & Khairuddin, N. (2009). Structural characterization and physical properties of antimicrobial (AM) starch-based films. *World Academy of Science, Engineering and Technology*, 55, 432–440.

Sattar, S. A., & Tetro, J. A. (2001). Other food-borne viruses. In: Hui, Y. H., Sattar, S. A., Murrell, K. D., Nip, W. K., & Stanfield, P. S. (Eds.), *Food-Borne Disease Handbook, Viruses, Parasites, Pathogens, and HACCP*, 2nd ed., vol. 2. Marcel Dekker, New York, pp. 127–136.

Splane, E. C., Rowland, N. E., & Mitra, A. (2019). *Psychology of Eating: From Biology to Culture to Policy*. Routledge.

Su, X., Li, X., Li, J., Liu, M., Lei, F., Tan, X., ... & Luo, W. (2015). Synthesis and characterization of core–shell magnetic molecularly imprinted polymers for solid-phase extraction and determination of Rhodamine B in food. *Food chemistry*, 171, 292–297.

Suara, R. O., & Crowe Jr, J. E. (2004). Effect of zinc salts on respiratory syncytial virus replication. *Antimicrobial Agents and Chemotherapy*, 48(3), 783–790.

Tallon, L. A., Love, D. C., Moore, Z. S., & Sobsey, M. D. (2008). Recovery and sequence analysis of hepatitis A virus from spring water implicated in an outbreak of acute viral hepatitis. *Applied and Environment Microbiology*, 74(19), 6158–6160.

Utami, R., Nurhartadi, E., Putra, A. Y. T., & Setiawan, A. (2014). The effect of cassava starch-based edible coating enriched with Kaempferia rotunda and Curcuma Xanthorrhiza essential oil on refrigerated patin fillets quality. *International Food Research Journal*, 21(1), 413.

Wang, B., Zhang, J., Cheng, G., & Dong, S. (2000). Amperometric enzyme electrode for the determination of hydrogen peroxide based on sol–gel/hydrogel composite film. *Analytica Chimica Acta*, 407(1–2), 111–118.

Warnes, S. L., & Keevil, C. W. (2013). Inactivation of Norovirus on dry copper alloy surfaces. *PLOS ONE*, 8(9), e75017.

Weingarten, H. P., & Elston, D. (1991, December 1). Food cravings in a college population. *Appetite*, 17(3), 167–175.

World Health Organization [WHO]. (2015). *WHO Estimates of the Global Burden of Foodborne Diseases*. [Access at July 21, 2020].

Xue, Y., & Xiao, H. (2015). Antibacterial/antiviral property and mechanism of dual-functional quaternized pyridinium-type copolymer. *Polymers*, 7(11), 2290–2303.

Zhu, F. (2021). Polysaccharide based films and coatings for food packaging: Effect of added polyphenols. *Food Chemistry*, 359, 129871.

4 Antiviral Biopolymers for Food Packaging Applications

Tannu Garg, Gaurav Sharma,
Rohit Verma, and Tejendra K. Gupta

CONTENTS

4.1 INTRODUCTION

During the 1850s, a British scientific expert made plastic orchestrated from bio-cellulose. Later, in 1970s, during the oil emergency in the USA, the biodegradable polymer acquired a great deal of significance. With innovations, now, various bio-materials are utilized as pure biomaterials in food packaging or mixed with glass, metals, and fuel-based plastic polymers [1]. Natural polymers are used as biopoly-mers often conveyed by living creatures. Biopolymers are the polymers which are identified as biodegradable. The intermittent rise of viral microbes represents a huge danger. The mass and bulk characteristics of a material are vital to at first build up material appropriateness for an application. The usefulness of many biomedi-cal devices depends on mass and surface properties, which can include both real

DOI: 10.1201/9781003243175-4

highlights and science [2]. It is possible to enhance current antimicrobial innovations and infection inactivation systems to promote antiviral products, which might provide an answer to this deadly contamination and food bundling. The SARS-CoV-2 pandemic (serious intense respiratory disorder), otherwise called COVID-19, spread internationally all through 2020 and has not yet seen an end. Notwithstanding SARS-CoV-2, a few viral pandemics, including the flu infection, human immunodeficiency infection (HIV), and SARS, have been reported in recent history. Inside food-related applications, these bio-based materials are especially valuable in three principal regions: food bundling, food covering, and consumable films for food and encapsulation [2].

Packaging is all items that are of any nature and utilized as the regulation, protection, presentation, and delivery of items from the unrefined components stage to the handled products and from the makers to the customers [3].

4.2 BIOPOLYMERS FOR FOOD PACKAGING

Biopolymers are the natural polymers that are produced from living organic entities. They are called "polymers" as they are made by rehashing a particular monomeric unit. The polymer from inexhaustible assets is expanding in popularity and acquiring consideration as a technique to create eco-accommodating materials. Materials that are used in the packaging of food are mainly recyclable or biodegradable polyesters, which can be taken care of by ordinary equipment. Some of these materials are at this point used in a couple of monolayer and multi-layer applications in the food packaging field. Based on the sources from where they are induced, they can be separated into four strands [4]:

1. The polymers are directly derived from biomass which includes proteins and polysaccharides.
2. The synthetic polymer is derived from biomass-derived monomers of oil-based polymers.
3. The polymers are produced by naturally or genetically modifying microbes.
4. The biopolymers are delivered through a compound combination of chemicals from both bio-based and oil-based monomers (see Figure 4.1).

An example of biomass-derived polymer derived from proteins includes soy protein, whey protein, and gluten. An example of biomass-derived polymer derived from polysaccharides includes chitosan, cellulose, and starch. PCL i.e. polycaprolactones, PVOH i.e. polyvinyl alcohol, EVOH i.e. ethylene-vinyl alcohol copolymers are an example of the second group previously mentioned.

The third group includes polyhydroxyalkanoates (PHAs) or bacterial cellulose. PHAs can be qualified by their complex underlying varieties, bringing about various properties and, consequently, various circles of utilization. Aliphatic polyesters are a crucial class of biodegradable polymers; various aliphatic polyesters have fabulous biocompatibility and biodegradability properties. There are numerous sorts of aliphatic biodegradable polyesters yet not a great many are financially

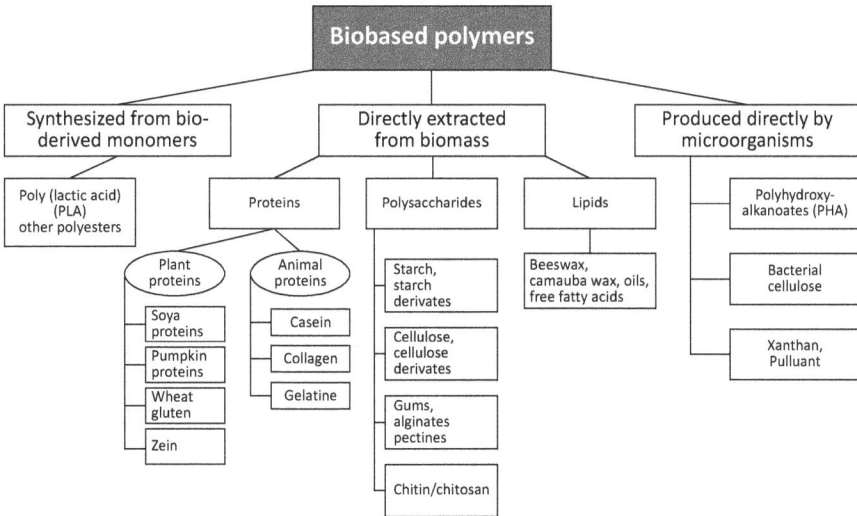

FIGURE 4.1 Classification of biopolymers depending on their extraction method [5].

feasible. The fourth group includes PBS i.e. polybutylene succinate, TPA i.e. bio-based terephthalic acid, and PTT i.e. poly trimethylene terephthalate. All of these biopolymers demonstrate explicit mechanical and designed properties that permit them to be utilized as a piece of the food packaging industry (Figures 4.2 and 4.3) [4, 5].

This large number of materials are applied in different mixes which also hold interesting unique properties as well as guarantee the quality, just as in the well-being of pressed food items. High quality and well-being are accomplished during the processing, handling, and storage of the item for the utilization of shoppers. This biopolymer gives a drawn-out utilization of food items additionally preventing any potential economic misfortune entailed by a significant food product [4]. For food loading, the elements of a food's connection with pressing materials and the surrounding conditions must be thought of. Materials that are utilized for food pressing ought to be equipped for giving ideal stockpiling of various food items. The plastics accessible in the market can be supplanted with comparative properties-based biopolymers which are petroleum-based.

These materials play an important role on account of the various environmental changes which can be an advantage for customers, financial specialists, and the producers of such products. Producing such materials is nevertheless a great challenge in science and industry [4].

4.3 COATINGS IN FOOD AND ANTIVIRAL ACTIVITIES

Some edible coatings are put on food to preserve and prevent the high quality of the food products. The active coating in foods are defined as continuous matrices which are prepared from natural and biodegradable food materials such as proteins, lipids,

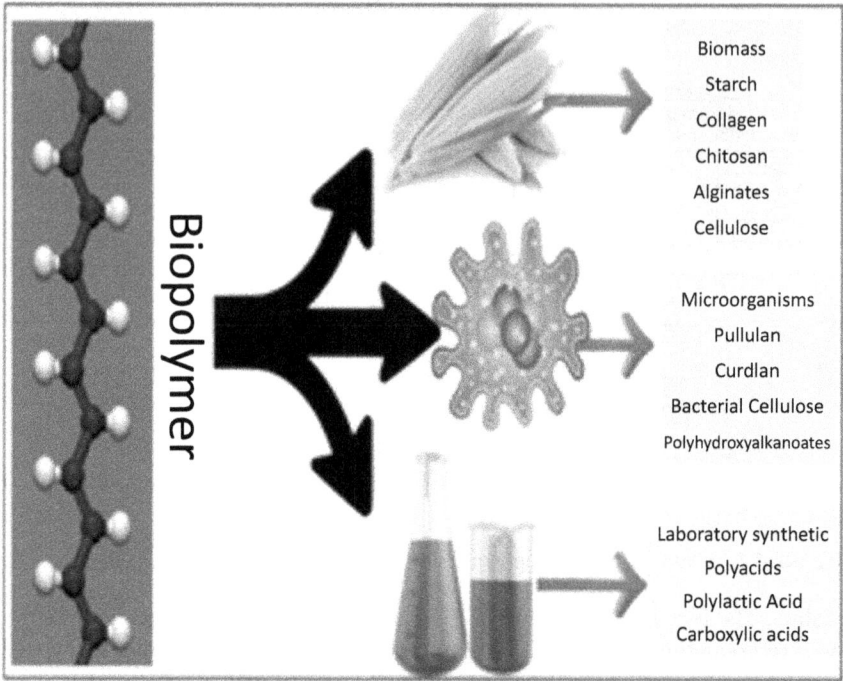

FIGURE 4.2   Cycle to produce biopolymers from natural resources [5].

or polysaccharides that support different functions depending on the specific product and its future anticipated properties [4].

The edible coating is used to prevent damage to food from moisture and gas and to improve its appearance and its storage life [4]. Additionally, an eatable covering applied should not deteriorate during cooking or utilization of the food item.

An ideal coating that can be used for food safety should satisfy the following characteristics [6]:

- An ideal coating must not contain any toxic or allergic components.
- It must be easy to digest or must not have any non-digestible components.
- It must stick to the food surface for the required time, therefore it should have good adhesive properties.
- A good ideal film should be easily manufactured and the economic value should also be taken into consideration.
- For an ideal film coating, there should be no loss of flavours or the nutritional or organoleptic characteristics which are needed for consumer acceptance.
- The aroma should not be lost while coating a food material.
- The film should be able to provide structural stability and should be able to prevent any mechanical damage during the transportation or handling of the food material.
- The coating should be able to provide microbiological stability.

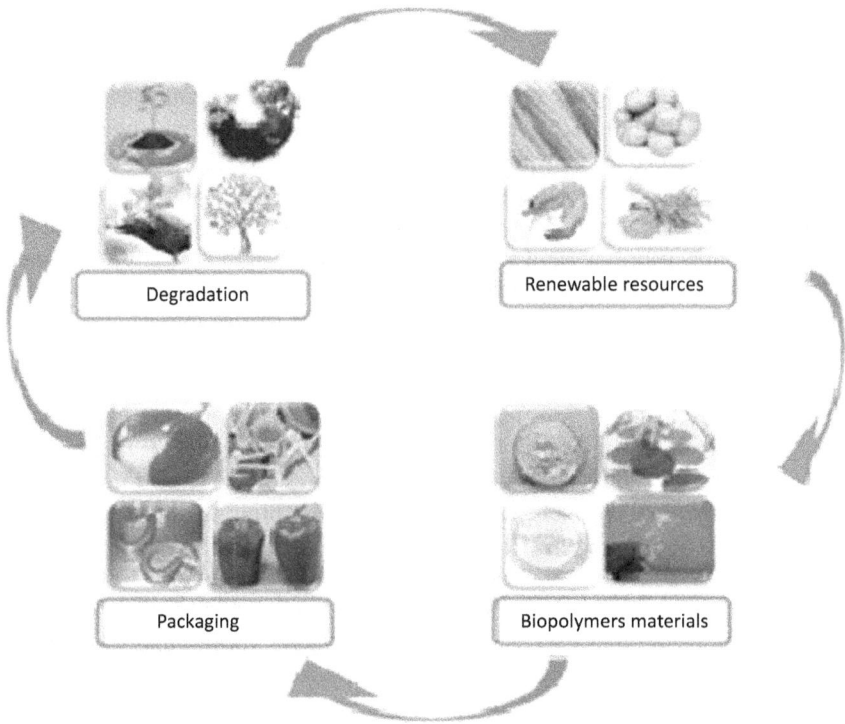

FIGURE 4.3 Representation of biopolymer from biomass, microorganisms, and labs [6].

- The covering utilized should give a semi-porousness so it can keep up with the inner balance engaged with the vigorous and anaerobic breath, consequently impeding senescence.
- The covering should have the option to improve the tactile characteristics (taste, appearance, and so on).

With the globalization of the food market and with the growing revenue for ready-to-eat food items, every one of these adds a test for the high-priority business to deliver a food covering which has the above attributes. A dynamic coating can be utilized, which can give help to the anticipation of transitory food sources. The counter microbial coating or antimicrobial coating can be utilized to restrain and kill the development of microorganisms by broadening the time-frame of the realistic usability of short-lived items and guaranteeing the security of bundled items [4]. There is an anti-oxidant coating that can be used in the covering which would then be transported into the food to safeguard it from oxidative degradation. Besides, the controlled appearance of these dynamic-dynamic combinations joined into packaging is relied upon to further develop the check limits in the creation chain.

4.3.1 STARCH-BASED BIOPOLYMERS

Starch is utmost in its abundance and is a sustainable compound in nature; it contains repeated units of ($C_6H_{12}O_6$) glucose and involves amylose and amylopectin. Starch has an exceptionally interesting substance and actual properties which are not quite the same as different carbohydrates. Starch can be gotten from vegetables, seeds, potatoes, natural products, and other items [4]. The polymers of starch are exceptionally sensitive to dampness and have extremely high water fume porousness and poor mechanical properties that limit their bundling application. Starch got from various vegetal sources gives polymer which can be utilized as the biodegradable polymer in food applications (Figure 4.4).

Starch is not a plastic material but a crystalline molecule structure. This crystallized form can be changed by the process called plasticization, in which the structure of its molecules loses its crystalline form and is converted into an amorphous form. The most innovative starch derived from this process is thermoplastic starch, abbreviated as TPS. This has the strong physical, chemical, and thermal properties of the final products. It is used to make bio-films, and bags, and used in lamination [4].

One example of biomaterial made from starch is PSM i.e. plastrach material, which is an exceptionally safe biopolymer. It is produced from plant starch and polypropylene with other natural modifying agents for various applications. It is a bio-based thermoplastic resin with extremely high water and oil proof, similar to traditional plastics. This additionally has high resistance from a variety of temperatures. Mater-bi is another starch-based plastic that is utilized to make items; such as shopping and waste biobags, and food administration things like plates and cutlery. BioBag is the world's biggest brand of certified compostable bags and films that have been produced using mater-bi [4]. TPS, abbreviation for thermoplastic starch, is made from corn starch which is derived from amylose

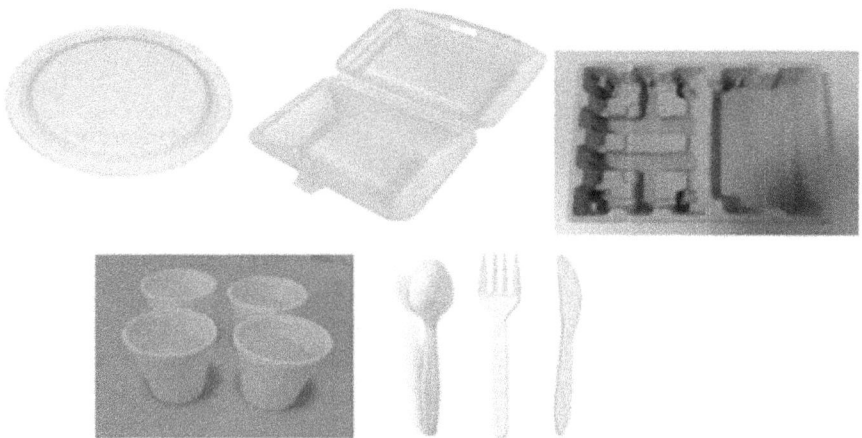

FIGURE 4.4 Biodegradable starch cups, plates, and cutlery [1].

molecule, which has exceptional compound properties which permit it for a wide scope of utilizations. Biomass bundling utilizes TPS to produce the water-solvent pressing material. The fundamental space of utilization of TPS is in food, restorative and drug packaging.

4.3.2 BIOPOLYMERS BASED ON CELLULOSE

The derivatives of cellulose are formed and they are commercially available in the form of methylcellulose, ethylcellulose, hydroxyl propyl cellulose, carboxymethyl cellulose, and cellulose acetate. Among every one of these, the most well-known and generally utilized food bundling material is cellulose acetate (CA). Cellulose acetate is characterized by low resistance to gasses and moisture and must be conducted through a plasticization process when used in the formation of films. Cellulose has a crystalline structure, due to which the first step when making its derivatives is quite difficult and costly. There are cellulose-based bio-films that are available, made from corn starch, soybean oil, and microcrystalline cellulose (MCC), which helps in the extension of shelf life by reducing moisture loss [4]. Cellulose to form films is quite expensive, which limits its wider industrial use. To produce an economically viable product made of cellulose, effective processing technologies for production have to be made. One of the business cellulose-based items is cellophane, which is a characteristic biopolymer got from wood. It is one of the very first biopolymers produced using cellulose and has primary parts acquired from trees and plants. This is produced from inexhaustible resources. This can be utilized as a packaging film for wrapping of bakery products such as pastry items, candy parlour items or other food wraps, or regular food-grade transparent bags. These films can have excellent oxygen, oil, grease, and moisture barrier characteristics (Figures 4.5 and 4.6).

4.3.3 CHITOSAN-BASED POLYMERS

Chitosan is a biopolymer that is utilized to make films that are solid and hard to break. They are more adaptable than petrol-based subordinates which are customarily utilized with comparative mechanical properties. However, they are effective as they don't have a lot of protection from stickiness and moisture. These chitosan-based materials have a low dampness hindrance, that causes it to have restricted use in food applications. Chitosan is not soluble in water yet it is dissolvable in acidic, citrus, and formic acids taking into account its cationic brand name. It has been praised for its antimicrobial, biodegradable, biomedical, and biocompatible properties and can be used in food and industry-related things to make chitosan a superior material for water fume penetrability. It tends to be joined with different polymers that make it steadier and precise to reduce into films. For instance, lipid and polysaccharide emulsions dependent on chitosan have been effectively utilized for dried natural product items and various kinds of cereals. New advances and mixes are executed to orchestrate and lessen the ineffective protection from moisture and water vapours of chitosan [4]. At Harvard, Wyss Institute specialists fostered a full degradable

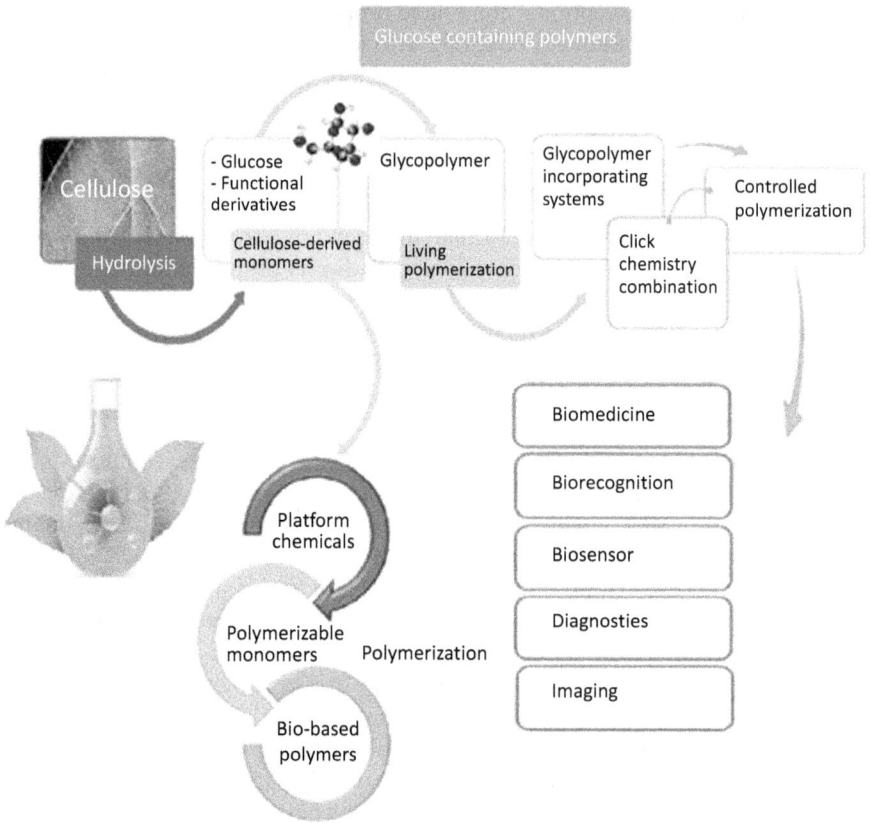

FIGURE 4.5   Process to polymerize cellulose and its application [7].

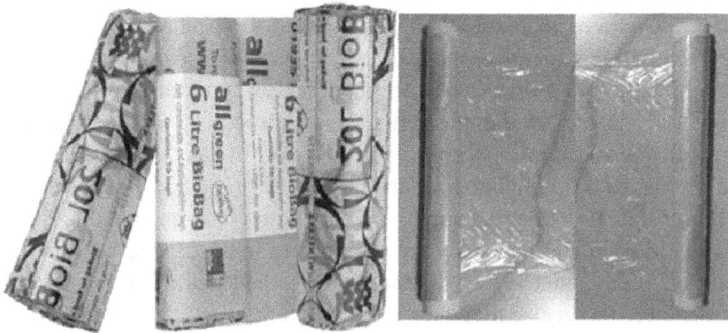

FIGURE 4.6   Biodegradable thermoplastic starch food gather sacks and cellulose films for bundling of various types of food [1].

biopolymer that has been disengaged from shrimp shells. This material then, at that point, can be formed into various shapes, as similar to conventional plastics without any environmental hazards. The chitosan biopolymers can likewise be utilized for the creation of various sorts of sacks, and food packaging in various shapes, while delivering rich supplements that are appropriate for the development and development of plants [7]. Chitosan is non-harmful, biodegradable, and biocompatible; along these lines, a harmless solution is considered for the ecosystem material for bundling. Dynamic bundling is an inventive way to deal with and further develop the timeframe of realistic usability of food while working on quality, respectability, and well-being (Figure 4.7).

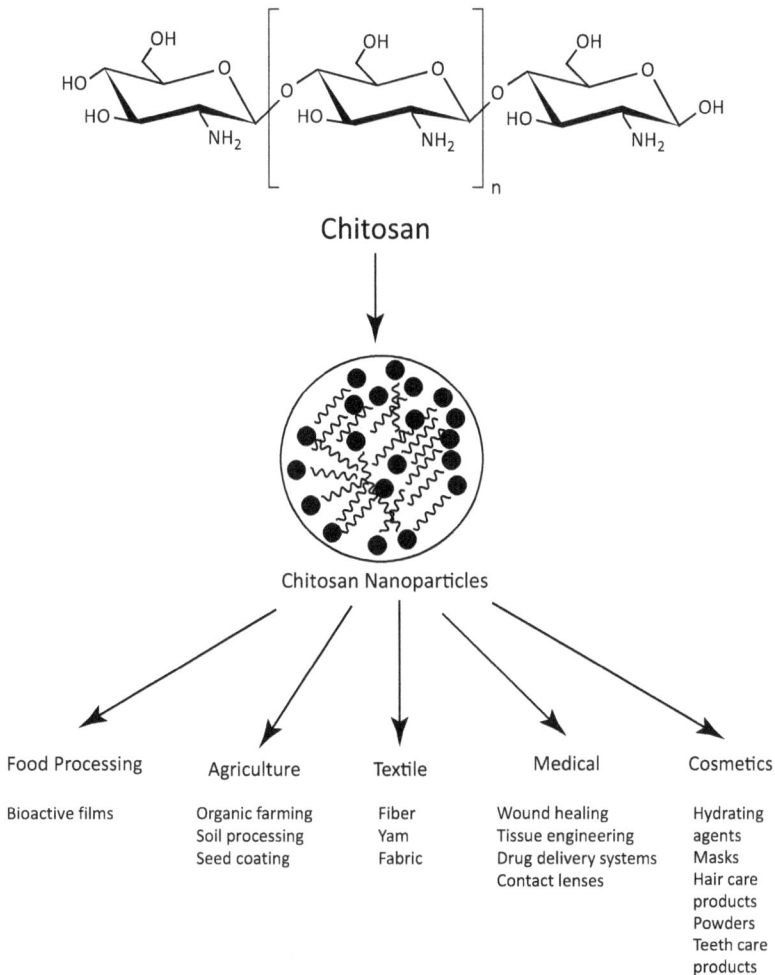

FIGURE 4.7 Structural representation of a chitosan compound form and its applications [2].

4.3.4 POLYLACTIC- (PLA-)BASED POLYMERS

The PLA, for example, polylactic acid, is a thermoplastic that is a biodegradable and inexhaustible biopolymer. This is got from the polymerization of the lactic corrosive monomer. Lactic acid is an essential monomer that is acquired from bacterial maturation of polysaccharides or through synthetic synthesis [3]. This can be an unmistakable option in contrast to petroleum and chemical-based plastic, like PS (polystyrene) and PET (polyethylene terephthalate). By and large, it tends to be utilized to make take-out packaging, covered paper, beverage cups, different cups, and new packaging.

For the development of biopolymer of PLA, the main fundamental monomer unit is the monomer of lactic acid which after polymerization forms PLA. The PLA has an extremely high potential for application as it would go about as an exceptionally clean bundling material for the food business. The most normally utilized polymer is possibly 90% L-lactide and 10% racemic D, L-lactide in packaging applications. By creating this material, it tends to be polymerized, dissolved, and effortlessly arranged. The PLA composite which is acquired through changing the polymer with 2-methacryloyloxyethyl isocyanate (MOI) has fundamentally worked on the physical, mechanical, and warm properties of the last biopolymer. This MOI polymer is exposed to a higher level of extending than the unadulterated type of PLA [4].

PLA in a copolymerized structure with other bio-polyesters has further developed the actual properties fluctuate altogether. The PLA polymers are generally recognized as safe, and in this way, it is allowed to be utilized in direct food contact with different food, for example, watery, acidic, and greasy food under the temperature of 60°C. The high elastic modulus and low hardness are the physical properties of PLA that are similar to polystyrene. PLA in its amorphous structure is completely transparent, with outstanding thermal and physical properties. It is extremely adaptable and acceptable for an enormous number of uses, adaptable (for names, composites, and so on), or unbending and frothing (for food use) bundling.

PLA is utilized for packs of salad, spinach, fresh-cut fruits, vegetables etc. More than 40% of salad sacks and comparative materials for new food packaging have incorporated the utilization of PLA. The use of PLA in the packaging of processed and fresh food is generally preferred by several organizations to promote the sustainable and organic life culture. One such organization is Coca-Cola, which is investigating PLA for packaging [4]. They are presently utilizing a PET bottle that would contain around 25% PLA. Yet, this could prompt an issue that the container would become non-biodegradable and non-recyclable because of the mix of two fixings would divide a reusing level incomprehensible (Figures 4.8 and 4.9).

4.3.5 POLYHYDROXYALKANOATE BIOPOLYMERS

Polyhydroxyalkanoate (PHA) is another biopolymer-making material that can be made for food packaging as it acts as a barrier and protects the substance like customary bundling materials. They are biodegradable-based polyesters made up of alkanoic acids which may contain a hydroxyl group and no less than one utilitarian gathering joined to the carboxyl groups. PHA is another biopolymer-production

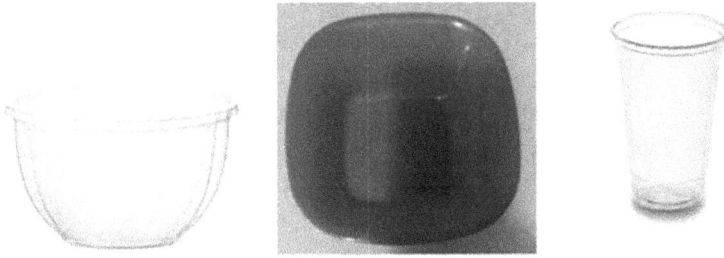

FIGURE 4.8 PLA-made cup and bowl [1].

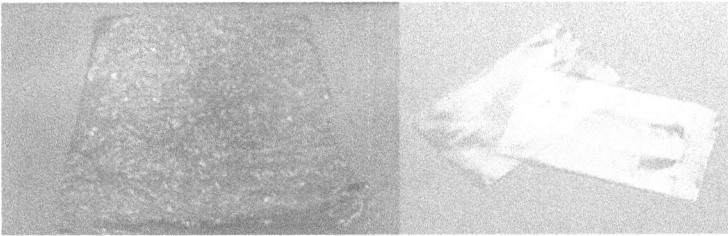

FIGURE 4.9 Polylactic acid (PLA) bags made from corn [1].

material that can be made for food bundling as it goes about as a hindrance and secures the substance like customary bundling materials.

The PHAs have oxygen and ultraviolet light resistance. PHAs with different polymers can possess different properties depending upon their chemical composition. They have a water-soluble nature with high surface energy so they are mainly suitable for printing and dyes. PHA is utilized as an adaptable food bundling with high oil content or frozen food sources. The PHAs can be inserted in the network of biomaterials which can be made into bio-coatings, covers, and biodegradable colour printing. The business utilization of PHA items dispatched on the market was for expulsion covering and cast films [4].

PHAs are regular materials whose life cycle is inexhaustible, as it is delivered and gets deteriorated by microorganisms. Thermoformed cups have been formed by using PHA resins. These cups have good stiffness and tensile strength like polypropylene cups. The PHA resin is made from aliphatic polyesters, which are made biologically by the conversion of the product of photosynthesis using microorganisms. The raw materials for its production are corn and other sugars such as carbohydrates (Figures 4.10 and 4.11).

4.4 GROWTH OF FOOD-GRADE BIOPOLYMERS HAVING ANTIVIRAL ACTIVITY

Food-grade biopolymers are used as an application for antimicrobial packing. This directly links to food safety and also helps increase the shelf life by prohibiting the progress of pathogens and microbes thus preventing the spoilage of food [8].

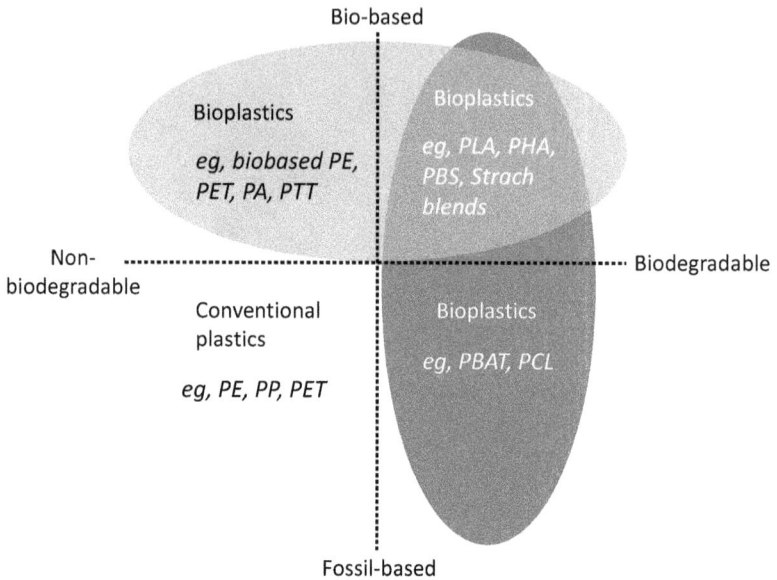

FIGURE 4.10 Representing the bioplastic PLA, PHA as a biodegradable alternative over petroleum-based plastic [9].

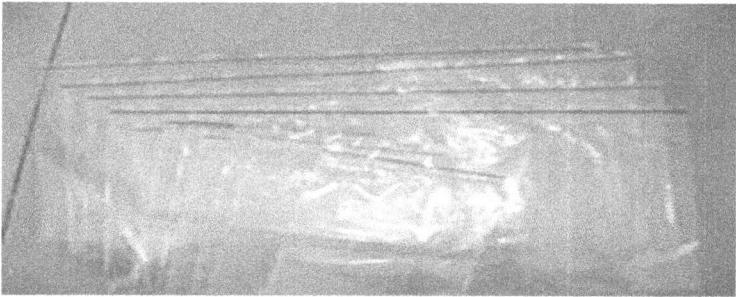

FIGURE 4.11 Various types of PHA bags are used for packaging [1].

Various biopolymer matrices are used and they serve as excellent carriers for an antimicrobial agent. Various studies show the antimicrobial effectiveness of essential oils and natural extracts. Bactericide and fungicide can be easily studied in comparison to antiviral activities. There is just a little information about the antiviral nature of biopolymers. Biopolymers can behave as antiviral agent in different fields such as food packaging, edible coatings, and contact surfaces.

New processing methods with better equipment and conditions are developed for casting and melting the compound to form new packaging functionalities that are the antiviral coating. The antiviral compound's effectiveness can be enhanced by developing a multi-layer structure that encapsulates the active compound and also modifies the biopolymer surface which can be increased with an increase in viral activity [8].

Antiviral polymers for food application can be made by:

1. Food contact surface. 2. Active packaging material. 3. Coating. 4. Encapsulation (Figure 4.12).

The polymer that can be used to make food contact surfaces is PLA (polylactic acid) and PHBV (hydroxybutyrate-co-3-hydroxyvalerate) with an active compound of silver and copper nanoparticles. PLA, PHBV(hydroxybutyrate-co-3-hydroxyvalerate), and chitosan are used to make active packaging material with active compounds of silver and GTE (green tea extract). Coatings can be made of alginate and encapsulation can be done by chitosan. Antiviral materials are available for food contact surfaces. The infection, whether viral or bacterial in an individual is spread through contact starting with one individual and then onto the next or through contaminated food or water, and protection from synthetic inactivation make human intestinal infections profoundly contagious through ecological fomites, including food contact surfaces. Normal areas and offices, for instance, emergency clinics, journey boats, cafés, and shared kitchens, are affected by such viral hazards.

Different surfaces like nonporous which incorporate glass, tile, plastic, polystyrene, treated steel, aluminium, and permeable surfaces like fabric produced using cotton, papers are accounted for as having intestinal viruses [8].

Reasonable and sustainable polymers have also been used for exemplification purposes. Exemplification has as of late been portrayed as a development to achieve sensitive substances' protection from the effects of hostile conditions. The term "microencapsulation" implies a portrayed methodology for wrapping solids, liquids, or gases in little holders, which can convey their substance under express conditions (Figure 4.13) [6].

4.4.1 Coatings and Active Coatings in Foods

With the globalization of the food market and with the expanding interest for ready-to-eat items with negligibly handled food the bundling business has a ton of difficulties. Dynamic covering is one such technique that can be utilized to help the protection of transient food sources. This dynamic covering goes about as an antimicrobial covering that can kill or hinder the development of microorganisms subsequently securing and broadening the period of usability of short-lived items and guaranteeing the well-being of bundled items. Keeping in mind the request to supply antioxidant coatings into the food to protect it from oxidative debasement can likewise be useful in ensuring nourishment for a more drawn-out time frame. Moreover, the controlled arrival of these dynamic mixtures fused into bundling is expected to upgrade the hindrance capacities in the creation chain. The expanding interest in eatable films and coatings is because of their capacity to fuse an assortment of utilitarian fixings. For instance, plasticizers, like glycerol, polyethylene glycol etc are regularly used to change the mechanical properties of the film or covering. The

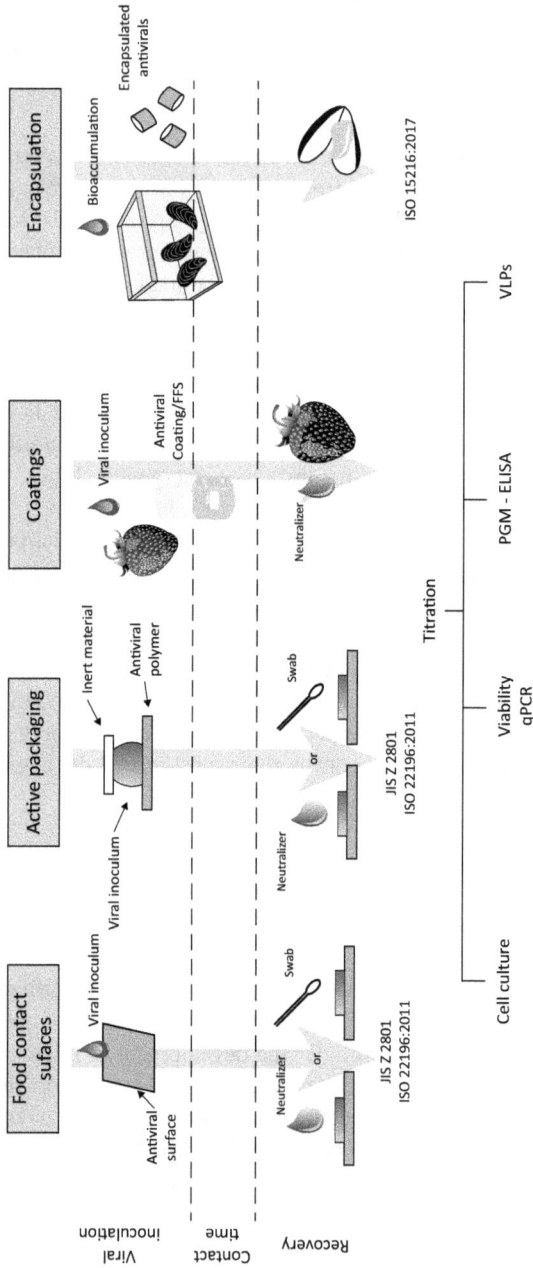

FIGURE 4.12 Chart of the strategies utilized for evaluating the antiviral movement of food-grade polymers or biopolymers [8].

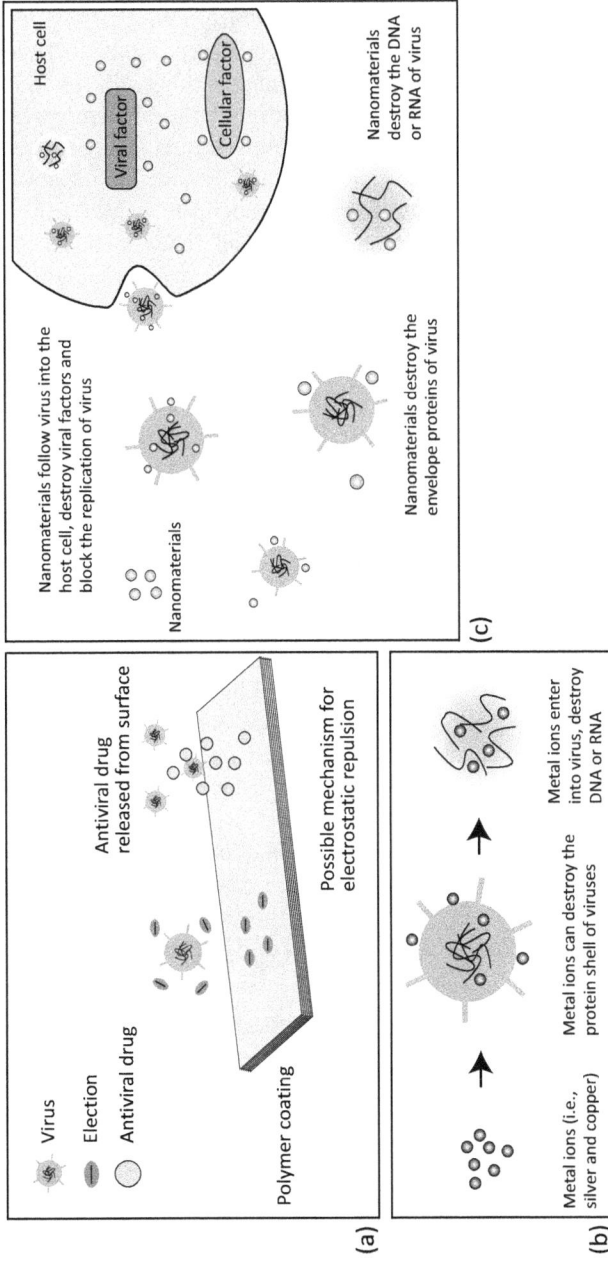

FIGURE 4.13 Diagram representation of the antiviral coating by different materials: (a) polymer coatings; (b) metal ions; (c) functional nanomaterials [2].

trading of smell compounds into the packaging changes the organoleptic properties of the food during the limit. A new investigation is also being coordinated into the possible utilization of nanoparticles in to consumable films and coatings [6].

Applying consumable coatings by dipping an object into, brushing, or giving it an answer containing film trims may be the easiest approach to do it. Thus, depending upon the proportion of the covering game plan, the thing will hold a reasonable proportion of covering material essential to outline the ideal cautious layer at the food surface, when dried. A such formed single polymer part is consistently incredibly sensitive and delicate. A few plasticizers should be added to the covering solution to prevent the producing coatings from getting delicate in order to maintain the covering. The plasticizer–polymer extent is the best approach to choosing the useful properties of coatings. Materials like sucrose, sorbitol, mannitol, and glycerol can be used as food-grade plasticizers. Given that its most pleasant components undergo fundamental changes at high temperatures, a thermo-plan is rarely used to create consumable films or coatings.

Chitosan is one of the biomaterials which is a potential threat to microbial properties and can be utilized as a bundling specialist to protect food against a wide assortment of microorganisms. Many investigations have demonstrated the adequacy of the antimicrobial movement of chitosan when fused in other polymer networks. Joining antimicrobial mixtures into eatable films or coatings gives a clever method for working on the well-being and timeframe of realistic usability of ready-to-eat food sources. Some of the more regularly utilized antimicrobials incorporate benzoic corrosive, sorbic corrosive, potassium sorbate, lysozyme, lactoferrin, bacteriocins (nisin and pediocin), and plant-inferred auxiliary metabolites, like natural balms. regular antimicrobials which incorporate compounds and bacteriocins are most generally remembered for their connection to consumers' well-being concerns. Lysozyme is an illustration of perhaps the most regularly utilized antimicrobial chemicals in bundling material. It is a normally occurring catalyst and is viewed as successful against Gram-positive microbes.

Many investigations have shown the utilization of phenolic intensifies when present in teas, rice wheat, or natural products which showed an antibacterial impact. Meanwhile, restorative analgesics of oregano, thyme, cinnamon, lemongrass, and clove are among the most unique against strains of Escherichia coli.

4.4.2 Various Applications of Edible Coatings

These edible coatings contain exceptionally creative applications in the food business. These multi-part consumable films and covering have hindrance properties that rely upon their design and science and the communication between various film parts just as the encompassing ecological conditions [6] The edible covering enjoys the accompanying benefits:

- They prevent moisture loss.
- The edible coating helps in the formation of ice in frozen food.
- Increases the shelf life of the food.

- It can also prevent the oxidation of food.
- It helps in the movement of water vapours between parts of various water activities in a heterogeneous food framework.
- Work to oxygen or dissemination of carbon dioxide.

4.4.3 NANOTECHNOLOGY IN COATING EDIBLE BIOPOLYMERS

Nanotechnology and nanocomposites have given an exceptionally positive utilization in palatable films and coatings due to the expansion of nanoparticles that can work on their presentation. Different sorts of natural details, for example, cellulose-made nanoparticles or chitosan nanoparticles are used in recyclable polymer frameworks to upgrade polymer execution. Many experiments have been created which join microcrystalline cellulose nanofibers. Cellulose nanocrystals are exceptionally helpful for consumable bundling applications [6]. Various studies about dampness sorption and water fume porousness uncover that the expansion of cellulose nanocrystals diminishes the dampness partiality of hydrophilic films, which is extremely valuable for palatable bundling applications.

The controlled use and arrival of nanoparticles are significant for the drawn-out capacity of food varieties or for giving explicit advantageous qualities, like flavour, to a food framework. In any case, the literature notes that numerous vulnerabilities remain with nanomaterials, including the potential for bioaccumulation and humanoid well-being hazards. More investigations along these lines are needed to guarantee that nanomaterials are not a worry to human well-being. Nanotechnology for bundling is an expansion of the correspondence capacity of customary bundling and confers data to the shopper dependent on their capacity to detect, recognize, or record outer or inner changes in the creation climate [6]. Simple customary pressing is being supplanted with multi-useful clever bundling techniques to further develop food quality, because of the use of nanotechnology in this field. For food bundling material, new bundling arrangements will progressively zero in on food handling by controlling microbial development, deferring oxidation, and further developing an altered perceivability and accommodation.

4.5 ADVANTAGES OF BIOPOLYMERS

The pressing framework is utilized for planning products for transport, appropriation, stockpiling, retailing, and end-use. The item should have the option to be securely delivered to the end market in a characterized condition with reasonable expense. The regular oil-based polymers utilized for the development of various types of food bundles could be generally arranged by their application, practical properties in bundling, and substance of regulation in the bundle. These oil-based polymers, for example, plastic, are not environmentally friendly, lacking biodegradability just as their conceivable relocation into the food, which is one of the principal reasons they should be supplanted with biodegradable polymers [2].

Another advantage is that it requires less energy (up to 65%) to produce a biopolymer than to produce plastic. These plastics have a very long period for degradation which is costly as well as leads to huge environmental impact and contamination. For sustainable use biopolymers are the best materials that are safer than plastics as they have less toxic substances. Biopolymers save 30–80% in ozone-harming substance emanations and give a more extended period of usability than typical plastic. The extraordinary benefit of the utilization of biopolymers is the chance of consolidating nanoparticles that convey a few positive attributes, for example, hotness and cold dependability, non-porousness to gasses, strength, immovability, antimicrobial properties, non-penetrability to oxygen, etc [9].

The biopolymeric materials are biodegradable and are predominantly reasonable for the development of fertilizer, which conveys supplements and natural material to the dirt. The aftereffect of this, an expansion in water and supplement maintenance decrease in substance information, and anticipation of plant infections.

The starch or cellulose-based biopolymers show more than ten times more simple degradability than plastics. The burning of traditional plastics creates smoke and exhaust that are harmful to people, natural life, and the climate. It is not important to examine the incineration of biopolymers concerning their biodegradability over a brief period, yet were such cremation to occur, the vapour delivered would not be harmful to the climate.

4.6   PROBLEMS RELATED TO THE USE OF BIOPOLYMERS IN FOOD APPLICATIONS

The polymers made from a monomeric unit of cellulose and starch and also those made from PHA and PLA are naturally occurring and till now these biopolymers haven't been found to have any major health-related problems. The PHA materials are made ready from microorganisms which can be an issue of concern seeing as some strains utilized in their creation could be conceivably hazardous [9].

The physical and compound properties of biopolymers with their ecological effects determine the potential relocation pace of their fixings. Since these materials in a pure form can't be used (as their properties needed to be enhanced according to the demand), thus they need to be combined with other polymers. Unadulterated biopolymers (added substance free) generally have fewer properties than traditional ones. The additional substance migration rate from PLA and starch-based biopolymers were shown to be especially low. Regardless, these examinations didn't take into account the harmful limit of bio-nano-composites, considering the amazing arrangement of nanomaterials, even those got from a comparative bundle, and a shortage of recognized government-authorized testing conditions (Figure 4.14) [9].

4.7   CONCLUSION AND FUTURE TRENDS

From the current research that has been conducted it is very clear that the development of renewable biopolymers shows impressive results over the conventional plastic materials which are available on the market. With its eco-friendly nature, there is enormous potential in food-related areas; the materials can be generated with edible coating applications, as well as biodegradable packaging with active and intelligent

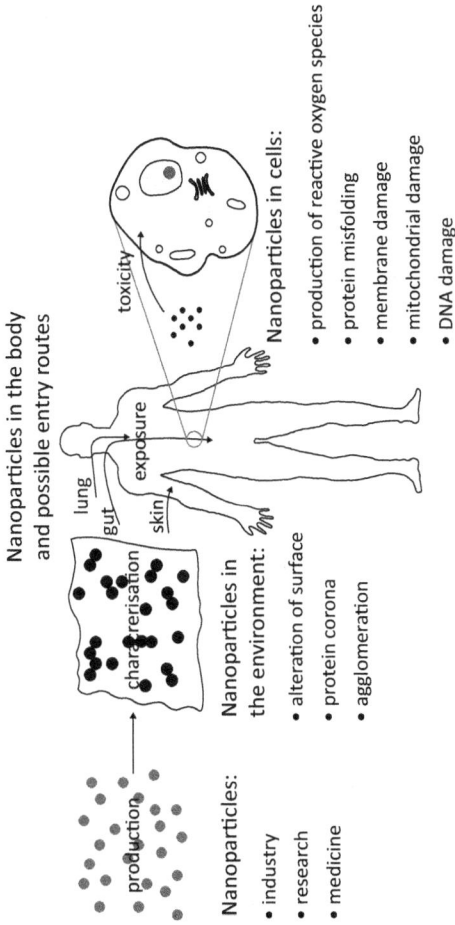

FIGURE 4.14 Impact of nanoparticles [10].

packaging [6]. To overcome some of their disadvantageous properties, especially as far as their hindrance execution, nanotechnology is currently being considered as a solution. Similarly, the innate assets of inexhaustible biopolymers are empowering the quick progression of the dynamic and the food packaging and embodiment encapsulation advances [6]. Different bottles, cans, containers, drums, vials, buckets, jars, barrels, terminations, covers, spray parts, food holders, bundling films, expendable cups, covering for assortments of bundling, bundling sacks, institutional and family reject packs, and crates etc are being delivered from decomposable polymers.

There is at present a wide scope of rigid property necessities for polymeric materials. These include [10]:

- Simplicity of handling and processing.
- Perm-selectivity.
- Low comparative moisture content reliance for obstruction to be compelling.
- Simplicity of reusing, or composability.
- More compelling obstruction properties to extremely durable gases, to dampness, and too low atomic weight natural mixtures.
- Brilliant chemical substance opposition.

With numerous antimicrobial mixtures making the polymers or composites, and nanoparticles which have been shown to work against bacteria, are hostile to parasites, or which are against viral action, they could be straightforwardly applied onto surfaces or consolidated into coatings to forestall the danger of spreading. Plastic is contained in many things that we buy. Part of the after-effects of artificial materials used in plastic packaging in an industrial context is that they are associated with substance aggravation, genital twisting, lessened productivity, and infection in a harmful form of energy which results in strong damage to the environment. However, regardless of the advantages, there are still a couple of insufficiencies, which hinder the broader commercialization of biopolymers in food packaging applications. The disadvantages are mainly a result of material execution and cost in comparison with standard materials, which remains a critical test for bio-based polymers. Regardless, it may require 20 more years to understand the potential outcomes of biopolymers used in food packaging materials. From now on, not all those involved in the local and national food industries should see the usage of bio-based polymers in food packaging as a mere decision but as a real need.

REFERENCES

1. Grujić, Radoslav, Dragan Vujadinović, and Danica Savanović. "Biopolymers as food packaging materials." *Advances in Applications of Industrial Biomaterials* (2017): 139-160.
2. Erkoc, Pelin, and Fulden Ulucan-Karnak. "Nanotechnology-based antimicrobial and antiviral surface coating strategies." *Prosthesis* 3.1 (2021): 25–52.
3. Adeyeye, O. A., et al. "The use of biopolymers in food packaging." *Green biopolymers and their nanocomposites.* Springer, Singapore, 2019. 137–158.

4. Fabra, M. J., A. López-Rubio, and J. M. Lagaron. "Biopolymers for food packaging applications." *Smart Polymers and Their Applications* (2014): 476–509.
5. Lisitsyn, Andrey, et al. "Approaches in animal proteins and natural polysaccharides application for food packaging: Edible film production and quality estimation." *Polymers* 13.10 (2021): 1592.
6. Popović, Senka Z., et al. "Biopolymer packaging materials for food shelf-life prolongation." *Biopolymers for food design. Academic Press* 2018. 223–277.
7. Shaghaleh, Hiba, Xu Xu, and Shifa Wang. "Current progress in production of biopolymeric materials based on cellulose, cellulose nanofibers, and cellulose derivatives." *RSC Advances* 8.2 (2018): 825–842.
8. Randazzo, Walter, et al. "Polymers and biopolymers with antiviral activity: potential applications for improving food safety." *Comprehensive Reviews in Food Science and Food Safety* 17.3 (2018): 754–768.
9. https://www.european-bioplastics.org/bioplastics/materials/.
10. Elsaesser, Andreas, and C. Vyvyan Howard. "Toxicology of nanoparticles." *Advanced drug delivery reviews* 64.2 (2012): 129–137.

5 Toxicology of Nanoparticle-Based Pharmaceuticals

Binu Prakash

CONTENTS

5.1 INTRODUCTION

Nanotechnology is a paramount innovative scientific area with enormous applications. New engineered nanomaterials and nanostructures have divergent properties and applications in different aspects of human life. Nanotechnology integrates diverse areas of science, engineering, and other fields of applied science, to produce materials with unique properties, such as high surface area, target sites, and slow release of specific elements (Ndlovu et al., 2020). The physicochemical properties of nanoformulations can lead to pharmacokinetic changes: absorption, distribution, elimination, and metabolism, which make it easier to cross the potential biological barrier, toxicity characteristics, and its persistence in the environment and human body (Soares et al., 2018). Nanoparticles may improve the stability and solubility of compounds, promote their transmembrane transport of them, and extend the cycle time, thereby improving both safety and effectiveness (Mitragotri et al., 2017; Kou et al., 2018).

The application of nanotechnology in the development of new drugs is now an emerging research field. Its use in medicine is called "nanomedicine" which is

DOI: 10.1201/9781003243175-5

defined as the use of various nanomaterials for the diagnosis and treatment of diseases (Tinkle et al., 2014). Nanomaterials can be applied to three different fields of medicine: diagnostic (nanodiagnostics), controlled administration of drugs (nanotherapy), and regenerative medicine. This technological development will make it possible to manufacture unique nanodrug compounds, which are used in the medical field, especially in the field of drug delivery.

The characteristics of nanomaterials have caused people to experience some adverse effects on their biological systems, especially at the cellular level. In recent years, different studies have been carried out that nanomaterials can affect the behaviour of organisms at the cellular, subcellular, and protein levels. More and more applications and products that contain nanomaterials or at least items that are nanobased are now available. The growing interest in nanoparticles used in advanced technologies, consumer products, and biomedical applications has not only sparked great interest in the potential benefits but has also raised concerns about possible negative effects on human health. Moreover, there is as well a far from systematic identification of nanomaterials in the framework of the authorization procedures for human drug development.

Nanomedicine which guarantees an advanced series of highly efficient compounds that can pass various biological barriers targets specifically the affected tissues. Besides, nanomedicine serves as an intelligent drug delivery system and a combination of both the diagnostics and treatment of a disease. There is currently no standardized protocol for describing the potential transformation of nanomaterials in biological systems. Therefore, it is time to check the significance of nanomedicine or other pharmaceutical applications and adverse effects (i.e., exposure, fate, and impact). The toxicological evaluation mainly faces challenges that include different definitions of nanomaterials and nanomedicine, different regulatory framework conditions, and the diversity of nanomedicine. This book chapter illustrates the different toxicological consequences resulting from pharmaceutically active nanomaterials.

5.2 NANO-BASED PHARMACOLOGY OR NANOPHARMACOLOGY

Nanodrugs that do not require the use of toxic solvents have obvious advantages over traditional drugs of the same kind. Several studies (Azimzadeh et al., 2017; Ramos et al., 2017) state that nanomedicine is likely to be a multi-component three-dimensional structure, and its function has thus far been preferred in a different area. According to various study reports (Blanco et al., 2015; Moshed et al., 2017), the application of nanomaterials is in surgery, cancer diagnosis and treatment, biological detection of biomarker identification, molecular imaging techniques, implantation technology, tissue engineering techniques, and also in drug delivery devices. Drug nanoparticles have been developed to control the release of drugs and protect it from enzymatic or chemical degradation to improve their therapeutic effect (Saeedi et al., 2019). Nanopharmacology focuses on the discovery of new drug entities, nano-level drug carriers, and drug selection, intending to use nanotechnology (as discussed in Figure 5.1) to selectively administer active parts to improve therapeutic effects and reduce toxicity. Nanomedicine includes very different compounds, species ranging

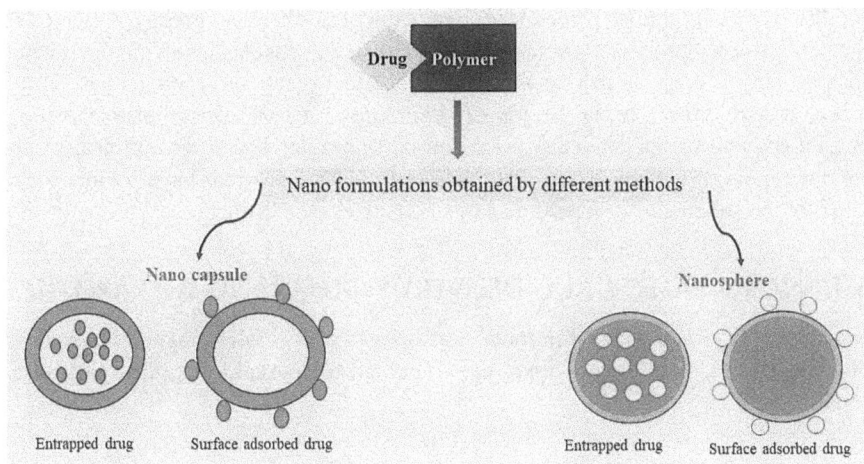

FIGURE 5.1   Nanoformulations of drugs.

from biological agents to abrasive products, liposomes, polymers, species of metals and metal oxide particles, species of dendrimers and quantum dots, and species of fullerenes and carbon nanotubes (Senjen, 2013).

   In the therapeutic field, drugs can be combined with particles/polymer matrices or embedded in the surface of the particles. Therefore, the demand for nanosystems in the medical field is increasing. The fate of a drug in the body is determined by various factors such as the drug delivery mechanism. An effective nanosystem for drug delivery must be based on the relationship between its biological system and the environment, target cell surface receptors, target cell population (Groneberg et al., 2006), mechanism, and drug site of action. The administration of multiple drugs and changes in cell receptors affect disease progression, molecular mechanisms, drug retention, and pathobiology of target diseases. Most research in the area of nanomedicine has focused on the development of new nanoparticle systems and the description of the physical and chemical properties related to their biological fate and function, especially in cancer diagnosis and treatment (Blanco et al., 2015; Stylianopoulos and Jain, 2015). Nanoparticle-encapsulated drugs exhibit different pharmacokinetics (for example, extended half-life) and better tumour targeting, leading to an increase in the use of nanocarriers in the field of medicine (Shuhendler et al., 2011, 2012).

   The local bioavailability of the drug administered by the nanoparticle is highly dependent on whether the nanoparticle can enter cancer cells and release its release or delivery at the site of action of the drug at a therapeutically effective rate (Meng et al., 2012; Ma et al., 2016). The cellular uptake of nanoparticles is a prime process of intracellular therapeutic drug delivery. According to the target site, nanoparticles interact with incompatible cell types after being administered in vivo. Pharmaceutical manufacturing of nanomaterials involves two different methods: top-down and bottom-down. The top-down process comprises breaking down bulk material into smaller pieces or smaller pieces using mechanical or chemical energy. In contrast, the bottom-down process takes up atomic or molecular species, allowing the precursor particles to upgrade in size by way of chemical reactions (Luther et al., 2008; Brandon et al., 2006). Initial attempts to gain knowledge of relevant pharmacology, physiology, and pathophysiology are essential to provide key criteria to design and estimate nanotechnology-based drug delivery mechanisms that have perfect functions for the treatment of several diseases (Zhang et al., 2018).

5.3   NANO-BASED DRUG DELIVERY SYSTEMS AND THERAPEUTICS

Nanotechnology is also used in molecular imaging, especially magnetic resonance imaging (MRI), fluorescence imaging, computed tomography imaging, and ultrasound technology.

5.3.1   DRUG-LOADED NANOPARTICLES

Drug-loaded nanoparticles impart a promising solution by selectively targeting tumour cells to avert damage to healthy cells (Misra et al., 2010). Biosensors based on the interaction of biological elements with nucleic acids are called biosensors or DNA biosensors or genetic sensors. Used to identify small concentrations of DNA (Moshed et al., 2017). The delivery of drugs to the injury site, as shown in Figure 5.2, is one of the key features of the drug delivery system and might be dependent on the efficacy of that therapy (Knight, 1981). Due to their better stability, nanoparticles are more effective drug carriers than liposomes (Fattal et al., 1991). According to Bamrungsap et al., 2012), several nanoforms have been analyzed as drug delivery systems, from biological substances (such as albumin, and gelatin) to chemical substances like various polymers and nanoparticles that contain especially solid metals.

Multifunctional response nanodrug delivery systems (NDDSs) are drug carriers with good targeting propensity, which is developed based on the first two targeting modes of the nanodrug carrier. In addition to the anterior targeting competence, this

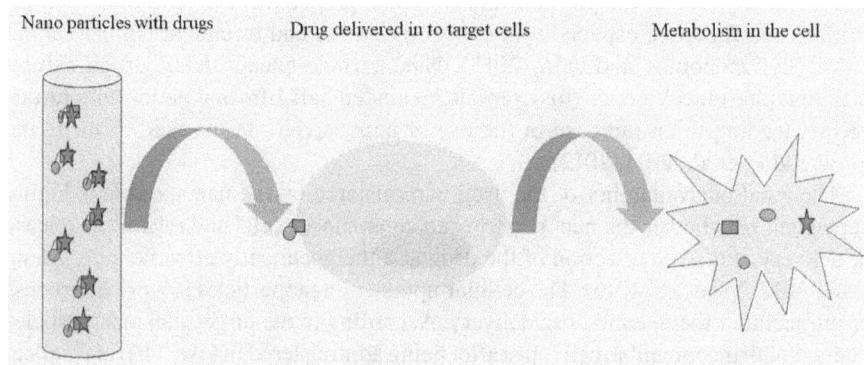

FIGURE 5.2   Nanodrug delivery system.

type of carrier is generally composed of reactive stimulating substances, which can be released from the special environment of the lesion under-stimulation, thereby reducing the release to normal tissues and increasing the accumulation of drugs. Diseased tissue. At the same time, diagnostic molecules can be assembled or labelled on nanocarriers to form an integrated diagnosis and treatment system. The ultimate goal of the clinical drug delivery system supported by nanotechnology is to upgrade the survival rate and quality of life of patients.

The Nano Drug Delivery System (NDDS) is used to encapsulate chemotherapeutic drugs and evinces excellent performance such as targeted delivery, tumour microenvironmental response, and site-specific delivery. A variety of nanocarriers have been approved for clinical cancer chemotherapy, and their efficacy has been significantly improved (Mu et al., 2020). NDDS can increase drug solubility and bioavailability, and extend drug circulation time through passive or active targeting. Figure 5.3 depicts various biological barriers involved in nanoparticle-based drug delivery. Moreover, it also dramatically increases the therapeutic drug accumulation in tumour tissues and enhances the area of pharmacokinetics. Nanoparticles loaded with anticancer drugs or therapeutic genes can use targeting moieties to target tumour sites. As we all know, compared to conventional non-targeted drug delivery

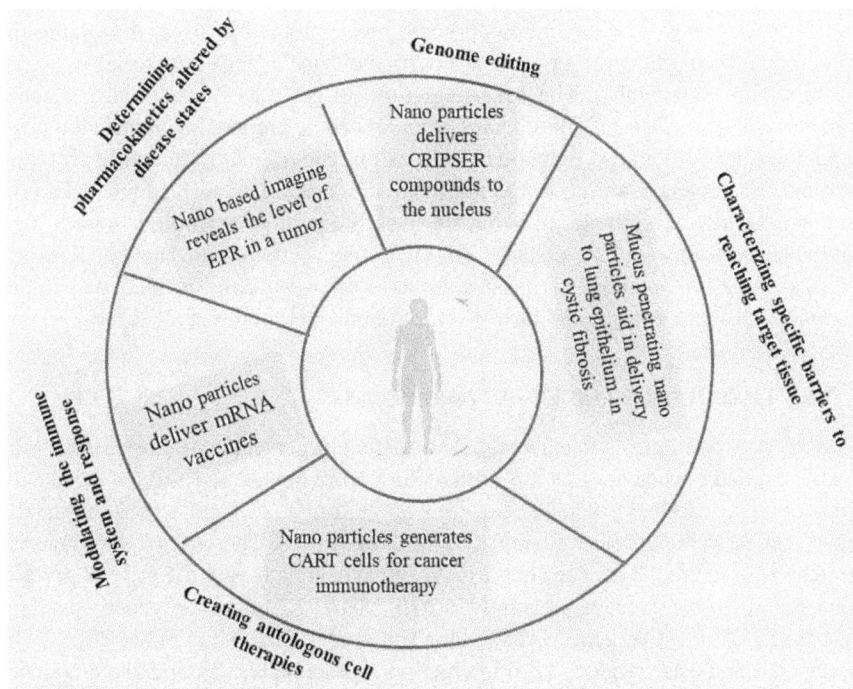

FIGURE 5.3 An overview highlighting some of the biological barriers of nanoparticles (NPs). Clustered regularly interspaced short palindromic repeats (CRIPSER); enhanced permeability and retention (EPR).

systems, targeted drug delivery systems can improve the therapeutic efficacy of their payload drugs.

5.3.2 ENCAPSULATION OF DRUGS WITH NANOMATERIALS

According to Whelan (2001), the encapsulation procedure is the foremost delivery choice for several drugs. The use of nanocapsules as drug carriers has much primacy. In the nano-encapsulation of drugs, drug-loaded particles with a diameter in the range of 1 to 1000 nm are created. Nanoparticles are defined as solid, sub-micron-sized active ingredient carriers, which may or may not be biodegradable (Couvreur et al., 1995; Reis et al., 2006). Moreover, encapsulation provides effective protection of the gastrointestinal mucosa, encapsulated in poly (lactic acid) nanocapsules, and also by reducing drug-related irradiation (Guterres et al., 2000). Nano-encapsulation of drugs/small molecules in nanocarriers (NC) is a very promising method for the development of nanomedicine. Modern drug packaging methods allow the effective loading of drug molecules in nanocarriers, reducing drug-related systemic toxicity (Kumari et al., 2014).

Emulsion polymerization is one of the fastest methods to produce nanoparticles and is easy to scale (Ribeiro et al., 2017). Depending on whether there is the use of the organic continuous phase or aqueous continuous phase, the process is divided into two categories. The continuous organic phase method involves dispersing the monomer into an emulsion or inverse microemulsion, or into a material in which the monomer is insoluble. The method is used to generate polyacrylamide nanospheres (Dai et al., 2019). Polymer nanoparticles can be prepared by interfacial polycondensation of lipophilic monomers such as phthaloyl dichloride and hydrophilic monomer diethylenetriamine in the presence and absence of surfactants (Jahangiri and Barghi, 2018). Alginate granules are usually made by extruding sodium alginate solution dropwise into calcium chloride solution. Chitosan nanoparticles are obtained by spontaneously forming complexes between chitosan and polyanions (such as tripolyphosphate), and have a small diameter (Carrillo et al., 2014).

5.3.3 GENE THERAPY AND DNA NANOVACCINES

Gene therapy is a technique currently used to treat or prevent hereditary diseases by modifying defective genes that are involved in improving the disease. Artificial cells are actively researched to replace defective or abnormal cells and organs, especially those related to metabolic functions (Orive et al., 2003). The goal of the antisense strategy is to interact with gene expression and avoid changes in the mRNA protein. Gene therapy is a technology currently introduced to treat or prevent genetic diseases by correcting defective genes (Maksymowych et al., 2002; Muul et al., 2003). The goal of the antisense strategy is to interact with gene expression and avoid changes in the mRNA protein. because of its ease of synthesis and direct functionalization of different residues, low immunogenicity, and toxicity (Muhammad et al., 2020).

The occurrence of new vaccines to deal with emerging diseases is still very important and one of the main goals of medical research. Historically, traditional vaccines, including live attenuated vaccines, inactivated vaccines, and subunit vaccines, have been very effective in treating infectious diseases (Zhang et al., 2017). Nanoparticles implemented as delivery vehicles protect the payload, be it vaccine antigens, proteins, drugs, or nucleic acids, from degradation in the harsh environmental conditions encountered during transport to target cells (Ramamoorth and Narveka, 2015). Due to their ease of functionalization, biocompatibility, and well-defined chemical properties, inorganic nanomaterials have attracted great interest in DNA vaccine delivery applications. In addition, its thermal and chemical stability promotes the sterilization process, which cannot be achieved with other kinds of materials (Liu et al., 2014). Nanomaterials have been studied extensively as DNA delivery vehicles and adjuvants due to their wide range of properties that can be adjusted by surface functionalization.

5.4 SIGNIFICANCE OF NANOMATERIALS IN HUMAN HEALTH

Over the past 20 years, the rapid development of nanotechnology has produced new materials that can be used for diagnosis and treatment. At the same time, there is an urgent need for the use of nanotechnology in the field of human health to improve our knowledge in the scientific field. Nanomaterials can improve the absorption of poorly soluble active substances by cells when delivering active substances. They also expand the bioavailability of effective doses of drugs that were previously difficult to achieve. Various studies (Weeraman et al., 2006; Zygmanski et al., 2013; La Spada and Vegni, 2018) also show that both the size and shape of nanoparticles play a significant role in the delivery of the drug. Nanodrugs can passively be transported to the cells, interacting simultaneously with the injury due to the presence of a large area of release. Nanomaterials can also be attached to different functional groups to address specific cells or stimulate the response capacity for the drug released (de Campos et al., 2004).

Over the past decade, nanomaterial-based drug delivery systems for the treatment of cancers have been extensively studied to improve the therapeutic effect and reduce the side effects of anticancer therapy. Since 2008, many groups have begun exploring graphene-based drug delivery systems. The surface area of graphene is higher, which allows it to be explored for drug delivery. Genaro et al. (2020) proposed another biomedical application. They pointed out that incorporating nano-hydroxyapatite into resin-modified glass ionomer cement (a restoration material) is a way to improve cell viability and tooth formation. The method of essential cell biocompatibility performance. The geometry of nanoparticles could significantly influence the rate of a load of drugs and the transport of drugs and the balance between dimensions and geometry is fundamental for the efficiency of the pharmacological administration (Ferji, et al., 2018).

Several nanocomposites for drug delivery have been manufactured using a variety of biopolymers and nanomaterials. The most common nanomaterials comprise nanoparticles of silver, zinc oxide, titanium oxide, gold, silica and clay, carbon nanotubes, quantum carbon points, graphene, and hydroxyapatite. In many studies (Lin et al., 2015; Ahsan et al., 2018; Martinez-Martinez et al., 2018), chitosan has been reported to be widely used in a variety of biomedical and pharmaceutical processes such as drug delivery, gene therapy, vaccine development, bioengineering, wound healing, and cosmetics manufacturing. Gu et al. (2013) designed closed insulin injection nanocapsules that were sensitive to glucose. The nanocomposites were composed of a chitosan matrix, glucose enzymes, and insulin. Chen et al. (2017) developed nanoparticles to deliver doxorubicin as per the demand in the cell. Doxorubicin was released by nanoparticles and was able to respond to both extracellular and intracellular pH values after injection into tumour-bearing mice. The nanomaterial-based vaccines are promised vaccine transport vehicles and enhanced specific delivery. Here also chitosan is a particularly attractive option for the supply of vaccines due to its very low immunogenicity, low toxicity, biocompatibility, and biodegradability.

The clays belong to a category of ingredients in the silica layers that are commonly used in the pharmaceutical industry, both as ingredients and in combination in compounds and hybrids. The nanotechnologist has designed several nanocomposites and hybrids performed with clay, which are based on the molecular structure and the physicochemical characteristics of the clay. Biopharmaceutical applications of nano clay are based on the help of the integration of the methods of release and engineering of the clay nanostructured in polymeric nanocomposites (Viseras et al., 2008). Biopolymer-clay nanocomposites (PCNC) have attracted great interest due to the wide range of edge properties compared to free polymers, such as greater mechanical resistance and maximum resistance to heat. The use of PCNCs for supplied medication purposes appears to be an interesting strategy to upgrade the characteristics of both clays and polymers. This is compared to the drug release mechanisms of the PCNC, the spread of drug molecules through the PCNC, swelling or erosion of the PCNC, and ion interaction between the drug molecules (Viseras et al., 2008). Studies have found that bio-nano particles made of peroxalate polymers can detect cancer (Sajja et al., 2009). This is because hydrogen peroxide is produced in human cells which have precancerous lesions.

5.5 CELLULAR AND TISSUE-BASED TOXICITY EFFECTS

The term "nanotoxicology" was first used by Donaldson et al. in 2004, they pointed out the fact that these differences require a special form of toxicology. Several studies have been made to estimate the effect of exposure to nanomaterials in human cell lines and other mammals. Morphology, shape, and structure are other factors that play an important role in nanoparticles' toxicity. The indirect estimation of exposure to the nanomaterials on human health can be evaluated by the analysis of the effect of the nano-based particles on these biological organisms. In recent years, many government agencies in various countries have begun to fund toxicological research to combat the potential dangers of nanoparticles. At present, research in the field of nanomedicine is, on the whole, focused on the application of nanotechnology (Zhao and Castranova, 2011). Product development generally does not consider the systematic toxicological evaluation of these nanomaterials.

Nanotoxicological studies have shown that the toxicity of nanomaterials is inversely proportional to particle size. Several studies have shown that these nanoparticles have

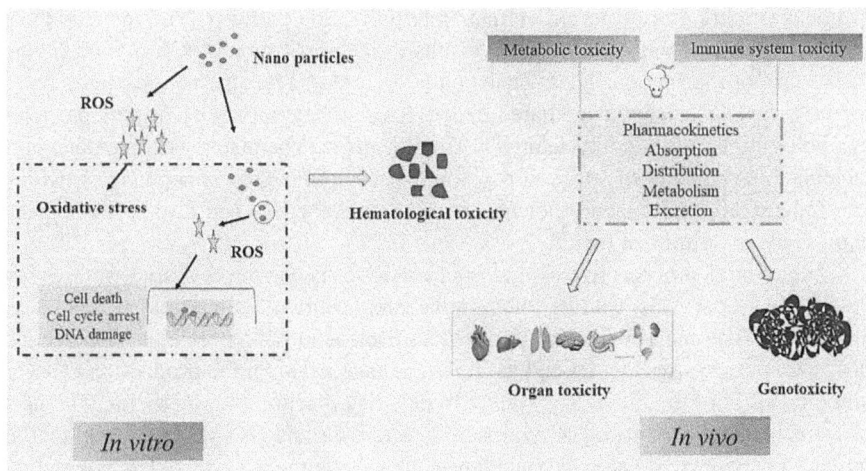

FIGURE 5.4 Cellular and tissue level toxicity caused by nanomaterials.

different toxicity characteristics from larger particles. Nanotoxicology is defined as a branch of bio-nanoscience that evaluates the toxic effects of nanomaterials/particles on organisms and other biological systems (Ai et al., 2011). Myllynen et al. (2008) discovered the essence of the nanotoxicology problem. Hagens et al. (2007) investigated the dynamics of nanoparticles in vivo.

The interaction of nanoparticles with the soft surfaces of biological systems plays an important role in their biomedical function and toxicity, as shown in Figure 5.4. To discover or design new biomedical functions or predict the toxicological consequences of nanoparticles in the body, it is necessary to understand the interaction process between nanoparticles and target cells (Xia, 2008; Vallet-Regi and Tamanoi, 2018). Once the nanoparticles are assimilated, if they can enter the cycle, they can be delivered throughout the body. For particles of reduced size, the ratio between the relative surface area and their volume (or mass) will increase rapidly. Since this surface can interact with the biological components of the cell, the reactivity of nanoparticles towards larger particles can be elevated (Brown et al., 2001). When nanoparticles enter the circulation, they can interact with blood elements such as plasma proteins and other factors that affect coagulation. However, the exact mechanism of this interaction is unclear. Evidence shows that the interaction of nanoparticles with plasma protein can reduce its toxicity. In vitro and in vivo studies show that compared with other forms of carbon nanoparticles, these nanoparticles have higher biocompatibility and lower toxicity (Wierzbicki et al., 2013; Zindler et al., 2016).

The degree of intracellular uptake of nanoparticles describes their cytotoxicity. For example, gold nanoparticles (cationic) are cytotoxic while anionic nanoparticles somehow are not (Goodman et al., 2004). Nanoparticles that are small enough can enter the circulatory system from the lungs and become systemic. In 2015, Haliullin et al. reported that the nanomaterials designed have toxic effects on fibroblasts and epidermal keratinocytes and, furthermore, may alter the gene or protein. Each type of nanoparticle has a preferred cellular internalization pathway. The incubation of gold nanoparticles with cells usually results in the adsorption of serum proteins on the surface of the nanoparticles. Zhao et al. (2011) stated that the nanoparticles enter the cells through receptor-mediated endocytosis. The cytotoxicity of nanoparticles can be easily annihilated by relatively simple surface chemistry. For example, surface chemistry has been successfully applied to modify gold nanoparticles, which can functionally refine the efficiency of gene delivery and can also regulate gene expression and diminish toxicity.

The production of reactive oxygen species (ROS) is one of the main toxic mechanisms of nanoparticles, leading to oxidative stress, inflammation, lipid peroxidation and protein, cell membrane, and deoxyribonucleic acid (DNA) damage (Fard et al., 2015). Oxidative stress is defined as the imbalance between the production of ROS and the ability of the biological system to detoxify reaction intermediates. The new physicochemical properties of engineered nanomaterials (ENM) make a potential target for phagocyte uptake and interaction with the immune system. The interaction of ENM with phagocytes, lymphocytes, and mast cells produced a variety of adverse reactions, including inflammation, immune regulation, and hypersensitivity (Smith et al., 2018). Toxicology and epidemiological studies have shown that the toxicity of nanoparticles depends on many of the physicochemical properties and exposure conditions of the nanoparticles.

Small inferring RNAs (siRNAs) have great therapeutic potential in the treatment of various genetic diseases, from cancer, viral infections, and neuropathy to different autoimmune diseases. siRNA nanocarriers for the process of systemic transport have been made to encapsulate siRNA, which are kept in the same form in the circulation, then finally transport the siRNA payload to the cell which is targeted. Then they interact with the cell surface, enter the cell, and effectively leave the endosome-lysosome system to remove siRNA is released into the cytoplasm (Kesharwani et al., 2012; Zhao et al., 2013). In the circulation, nanoparticles are taken up primarily by mononuclear phagocytes as a storage and defence mechanism. The rate of this uptake is the determinant of the half-life of nanoparticles in the blood. Some circulating proteins (such as opsonins) bind to nanoparticles in the blood and increase the rate of phagocytosis (Landsiedel et al., 2012). The vascular endothelium with tight junctions is the next barrier for nanoparticles to enter cells. The distribution of nanoparticles in organs mainly turns out in the liver, followed by the spleen, lymph nodes, and bone marrow (Sahay et al., 2010; Landsiedel et al., 2012). Some nanoparticles can cross the blood-brain barrier, and this absorption can be facilitated by negative surface charges and binding to proteins such as albumin. Figure 5.5 discussed the factors influencing the toxicity of nanoparticles in humans. The nanoparticles injected into the extracellular matrix can drain back into the circulation through the drainage of lymphatic vessels and lymph nodes (Vega-Villa et al., 2008).

5.6   POSSIBLE MECHANISMS BEHIND THE NANOTOXICOLOGY

Today, we have a better understanding of nanotoxicity based on our knowledge of how nanomaterials interact with biological systems. The actual range of exposure

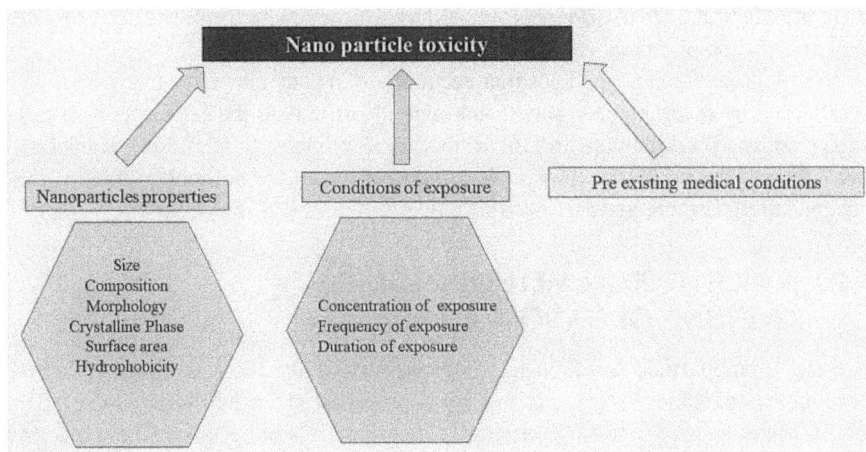

FIGURE 5.5 Factors influencing the toxicity of nanoparticles in humans.

to nanoparticles must be assessed, and the extent to which the toxicological data of larger particles of the same chemical substance can be used or extrapolated. Almost all toxicological experiments with nanoparticles describe an external exposure. External exposure sets out the total dose of ingested, inhaled, or applied to the skin nanoparticles. Internal exposure is part of the external dose of nanoparticles that reaches the systemic circulation and other organs and tissues (Hagens et al., 2007). Various research groups (Medina et al., 2007; Bakand et al., 2012; Lujan and Sayes, 2017) have studied the cellular response and toxicological pathways of nanoparticles interacting with cells. Experimental results show that the main cellular responses of nanoparticles include antioxidant response, pro-inflammatory effects, lysosomal generation, mitochondrial membrane potential reduction, calcium release, caspase activation, cell apoptosis, and cell death (Zhao et al., 2011).

Various extrapolations may require sufficient information on the absorption, distribution, metabolism, and excretion (ADME) of nanoparticles. In addition to the toxicological studies of nanoparticles, additional "case-by-case" toxicokinetic studies on disparate types of nanoparticles are required to ensure their safe use.

Once the nanoparticles are absorbed by the gastrointestinal tract, these particles are transported directly to the liver through the portal vein. The liver can actively separate compounds from the blood. In addition, nanoparticle drug delivery systems made of liposomes can fuse with the plasma membranes of the cell. The drug let out in the cell can be metabolized consequently to the normal metabolic pathway set out in the conventional drug preparation. There are diverse kinds of mechanisms for the removal of particles from the lungs (external exposure), or the systemic removal of nanoparticles (internal exposure). Nanoparticles absorbed in the body's circulation can be excreted from the body in many ways. Kidney clearance may be a possible way to eliminate nanoparticles (Zuckerman et al., 2012). Similar to common chemicals, the dose of nanoparticles at the target point in the body plays a decisive role in the observed effects. To obtain information about the dose of nanoparticles (in vivo), there is an urgent need to develop validated (real-time) methods for the detection and characterization of nanoparticles in biological fluids and tissues.

Non-degradable nanoparticles that accumulate in cells may have many effects. It is taken up by macrophages, it will undoubtedly stimulate the release of free radicals, leading to cell damage and inflammation (Kallinteri, et al., 2005). If nanoparticles are soaked up by the lysosomal compartment but are not biodegradable, they may accumulate there and cause toxicity (Garnett, and Kallinteri, 2006).

5.7 TOXICOLOGICAL METHODOLOGIES' PROFILING OF NANOMATERIALS

Although nanoparticle research has been underway for more than 30 years, the development of standard methods and protocols required for their safety and efficacy tests for human use is a work in progress. Therefore, it is important to meet the need for improved and standardized assessments of inorganic nanoparticles and the toxicity of various biomedical uses, for consistency of years between scientific developments and correspondents' health regulations and security (Hofmann-Amtenbrink et al., 2015). Humans and animals inhale, ingest, and absorb nanoparticles from the skin. After nanoparticles enter, they can damage cells and eventually organs through complex mechanisms (Fallah et al., 2021). Improvement of the methodology and test tools to distinguish research nanomaterials about trading versions and the life cycles of products are a necessity, to be prepared for unforeseen events and the potential effect of these materials on human health and the environment.

Nanomaterial products for industry and medicine should seek a common approach to security and toxicology tests. The measurements that use inductively coupled plasma spectrometry can be used to evaluate the transport and separation in vivo of animal nanoparticles (Abid et al., 2013). The in vitro evaluation method has received more attention in recent studies because of its lower cost, faster process, and minimal ethical issues. Common toxicity screening tests can be divided into in vitro tests and in vivo tests (Kumar et al., 2017). Sayes et al. (2007) measured the toxicity of nanoparticles with the aid of using evaluation for both in vitro and in vivo pulmonary toxicity profiles. After oral and intravenous administration in laboratory model animals, the biodistribution of nanoparticles of various geometric shapes, including rod-shaped, cylindrical, quasi-hemispherical, etc. were observed (Decuzzi et al., 2010). Nanoparticle toxicity in an in vivo model depends on dose and exposure conditions, duration of exposure, and route of administration (Love et al., 2012; Kumar et al., 2017). In vivo nanometre toxicity assessment experiments are mainly divided into six categories, including LD50 (50% lethal dose), serum chemical analysis, cell population, tissue morphology, histological studies, and a total of nanoparticle biodistribution and clearance analysis. The physical interaction between nanoparticles and deoxyribonucleic acid (DNA) may have potentially negative effects on their structure, stability, and biological function. Possible clinical outcomes related to DNA damage, especially cancers, may take a long time to be detected in the body. Therefore, the profiling method for studying the interaction between DNA and different nanoparticles may be very useful. Nanomedicine faces both safety and toxicological problems. In the case of the administration of nano-pharmaceuticals, these could be with the standardization of the dose of the drug, the dose required for clinical effectiveness, and the dose that causes side effects or undesirable toxicities. Nanoparticles have qualitatively different physicochemical properties from microparticles. Besides, the use of nanoparticles as an active ingredient carrier can reduce the toxicity of the incorporated active ingredient. In general, the toxicity of the nanoparticles' formulation as a whole is investigated.

Several current nanomedical products are based on reinforcement or adaptation of formulation strategies for long or insoluble soluble drugs with improved performance when encapsulated in lipid vehicles (liposomes) or as protein complexes, or in nanocapsules. The development of new tools capable of better detection of modifications required in the cells placed in contact with nanoparticles in a biological environment. Moreover, this includes methods for determining the number of particles in cell contact and interrogation of various cell signalling pathways simultaneously. Boxall et al. (2007) used a series of simple algorithms to predict probable environmental concentrations of a limited range of nanomaterials manufactured in land and water. For the water, the entrance paths included the following: direct Entry into water bodies; drift entries in the agrochemical spray; cleaning of contaminated land; aerial deposition. The difficulty with some of these approaches is to cover the full range of potential sources of nanomaterials and, as it is not a limited selection, we also need to reasonably estimate the use of the market. O'Brien and Cummins proposed a three-level model to determine the risk of exposure, starting with the establishment of exhibition concerns (level 1); determination of the characteristics of particles (dimensions, surface, surface change, solubility, etc.), behaviour (aggregation, adsorption), and treatment (level 2); and relating to exposure scenarios (level 3). This is sound, but trying to fill these levels with relevant data for the real environment again is difficult. Including the dosing algorithms in combination with information on the size of a nanoparticle, the procedure of application, and media would contribute to better defining the effects of these doses (Hofmann-Amtenbrink et al., 2015).

The focus of the field of nanotoxicology has recently shifted to understanding the details of accidental or undesirable interactions between nanomaterials and biomolecules. The application of silicon-based methods and methods to study the structural aspects of toxicity is related to the structure and dynamics of nanoparticles (Bedrov et al., 2008). One way to track the pharmacokinetics of medical nanoparticles composed of core and coating is to use dual radiolabelled compounds. There is currently no standardized protocol to describe the potential transformation of nanomaterials in biological systems. Metabolism and excretion in patient needs specific testing protocols. Information from in vivo toxicokinetic studies may help investigate whether nanoscale active substances are excreted. In 2017 DeLoid et al. proposed an integrated approach to blow up the impact of the food matrix and gastrointestinal effects on biokinetics and cell toxicity of engineered nanomaterial which is used in the food industry. A "standardized" research strategy for nanosafety with validated protocols and quality systems would therefore be useful for the development of new nano combinations. Figure 5.6 shows some of the toxicological kinetics for nanosafety. Apart

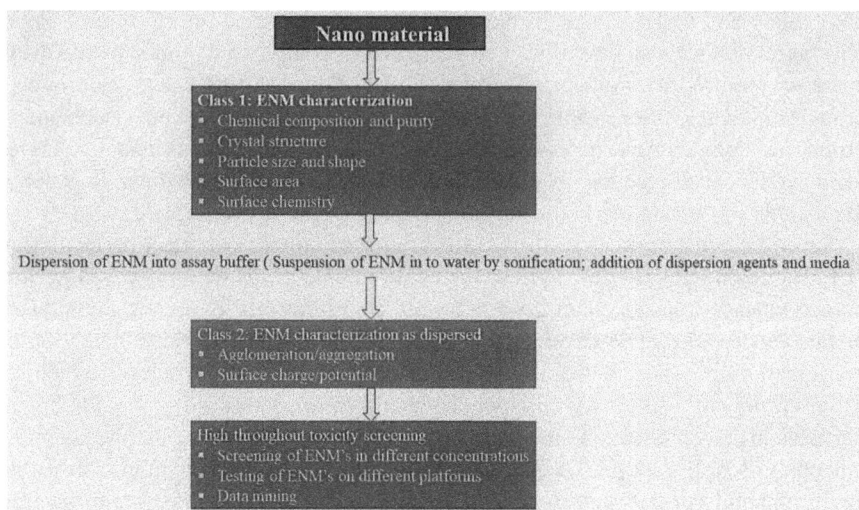

FIGURE 5.6   Kinetics properties of nanoparticles in the body.

from that, the problematical nanoparticle formulations could be recognized early enough to be eliminated.

5.8   ECOTOXICOLOGY OF NANOMATERIAL-BASED PHARMACEUTICALS

Due to the surge in applications and development, a large number of nanoparticles have recently entered the environment. However, one feature of nanomedicine is often overlooked: what happens after prescribed use and if nanomedicine residues eventually enter the environment. It is not difficult to envisage that the residue of nanomedicine or the nanomedicine carrier will have unexpected effects on the environment. Nanomaterials are very suitable for therapeutic purposes but problems may arise if nanomedicine is released into the environment. Researchers classify various nanodrugs to help address specific groups with specific demands for environmental risk evaluation. The clinical application of biodegradable nanoparticles and the safety of these nanoparticles have been improved due to the biodegradability of the nanomaterials used.

Environmental drug contamination has also been found in several states, such as groundwater sewage sludge, landfill leachate, or arable land irrigated with treated/ untreated sewage (Kummerer, 2008). It has been proposed that green nanoscience be used to reduce environmental and human dangers from the creation and use of nanomaterials and make advances in providing existing items with new nanoproducts that are more ecologically friendly (Iavicoli et al., 2014). Maiti et al. (2016) reported that the destiny of nanomaterials in the environment is controlled by the combined effects of their physical properties and their interactions with other contaminants. For nanoparticles, the issue is how to direct the relevant exposure concentration in ecotoxicology laboratory research and the environment; this is the result of preliminary hazard identification analysis. This makes it unfeasible to perform scientifically verified environmental impact and exposure assessments. Several variables may also act on the exposure assessment of nanomedicine, as well as changes in the characterization of the bioreactivity, size, shape, load, and route of administration.

Nanomaterials and drugs are steadily released into the aquatic environment and their concentration can vary between ng/L and mg/L (Balakrishna et al., 2017). The attachment of micro nanoparticles or MNP to the cell wall of microalgae restricts the movement of nutrients and energy in the external environment and brings down algae growth (Davarpanah and Guilhermino, 2019). The environmental risk assessment (ERA) of medical products for human use within the European Union (EU) is set on the guidelines for environmental risk assessment of medical products for human use. The ERA strategy for human drugs detailed in the Environmental Risk Assessment of Human Drugs was developed for small molecule drugs. When estimating the impact of nanomedicine on the environment, particular adaptations may be indispensable. The ERA of nanodrug products plays a decisive role in determining whether patients excrete nanoscale compounds and the number of nanoscale compounds expelled. When a nanoscale compound enters the body, a nanoscale-specific risk assessment must be performed. An important step is to recognize regardless the drug is controlled by or contains nanoscale compounds, which is requisite to prevail the comprehensive physical properties of the compound. This information must then be given in the environmental risk assessment module in the application file when seeking marketing authorization.

Batley et al. (2013) stated that the designed nanomaterials can enter soils through different sources and traces. In the environment, nanoparticles can undergo many possible modifications, depending on the properties of both the nanoparticles and the receptive medium. These transformations mostly involve chemical and physical processes but can involve the biodegradation of the superficial coatings used to stabilize many nanomaterial formulations. Most of the nanoparticles are hydrophilic and have a finite but often low solubility. The envisaged environmental concentrations of the nanomaterials manufactured in natural waters are types of less than 20 μg /L.

5.9 CONCLUSION

The multidisciplinary nature of nanotechnology has led to a large number of innovations, which poses a considerable challenge to the interpretation of cell and tissue toxicity. The toxicity of nanomaterials is of significance and a major problem globally, and because most of the studies in this field do not use the same method and standard, it is difficult to make comparisons. Therefore, the development and validation of toxicity assessment methods for artificial nanoparticles will be the focus in the future.

REFERENCES

Abid, H.R., Shang, J., Ang, H.M. and Wang, S., 2013. Amino-functionalized Zr-MOF nanoparticles for adsorption of CO_2 and CH_4. *International Journal of Smart and Nano Materials*, 4(1), pp.72–82.

Ahsan, S.M., Thomas, M., Reddy, K.K., Sooraparaju, S.G., Asthana, A. and Bhatnagar, I., 2018. Chitosan as biomaterial in drug delivery and tissue engineering. *International Journal of Biological Macromolecules*, 110, pp.97–109.

Ai, J., Biazar, E., Jafarpour, M., Montazeri, M., Majdi, A., Aminifard, S., Zafari, M., Akbari, H.R. and Rad, H.G., 2011. Nanotoxicology and nanoparticle safety in biomedical designs. *International Journal of Nanomedicine*, 6, p.1117.

Azimzadeh, M., Rahaie, M., Nasirizadeh, N., Daneshpour, M. and Naderi-Manesh, H., 2017. Electrochemical miRNA biosensors: The benefits of nanotechnology. *Nanomedicine Research Journal*, 2(1), pp.36–48.

Bakand, S., Hayes, A. and Dechsakulthorn, F., 2012. Nanoparticles: A review of particle toxicology following inhalation exposure. *Inhalation Toxicology*, 24(2), pp.125–135.

Balakrishna, K., Rath, A., Praveenkumarreddy, Y., Guruge, K.S. and Subedi, B., 2017. A review of the occurrence of pharmaceuticals and personal care products in Indian water bodies. *Ecotoxicology and Environmental Safety*, 137, pp.113–120.

Bamrungsap, S., Zhao, Z., Chen, T., Wang, L., Li, C., Fu, T. and Tan, W., 2012. Nanotechnology in therapeutics: A focus on nanoparticles as a drug delivery system. *Nanomedicine*, 7(8), pp.1253–1271.

Batley, G.E., Kirby, J.K. and McLaughlin, M.J., 2013. Fate and risks of nanomaterials in aquatic and terrestrial environments. *Accounts of Chemical Research*, 46(3), pp.854–862.

Bedrov, D., Smith, G.D., Davande, H. and Li, L., 2008. Passive transport of C60 fullerenes through a lipid membrane: A molecular dynamics simulation study. *The Journal of Physical Chemistry: Part B*, 112(7), pp.2078–2084.

Blanco, E., Shen, H. and Ferrari, M., 2015. Principles of nanoparticle design for overcoming biological barriers to drug delivery. *Nature Biotechnology*, 33(9), pp.941–951.

Boxall, A.B.A., Chaudhry, Q., Sinclair, C., Jones, A., Aitken, R., Jefferson, B. and Watts, C., 2007. Current and future predicted environmental exposure to engineered nanoparticles. Report by the Central Science Laboratory (CSL) York for the Department of the Environment and Rural Affairs (DEFRA), UK. wwTv.de-fra.gov.uk/science/Project_Da-ta/DocumentLibrary/CB01098/CB01098_627()_FRP.pdf.

Brandon, E.F., Oomen, A.G., Rompelberg, C.J., Versantvoort, C.H., van Engelen, J.G. and Sips, A.J., 2006. Consumer product in vitro digestion model: Bioaccessibility of contaminants and its application in risk assessment. *Regulatory Toxicology and Pharmacology*, 44(2), pp.161–171.

Brown, D.M., Wilson, M.R., MacNee, W., Stone, V. and Donaldson, K., 2001. Size-dependent proinflammatory effects of ultrafine polystyrene particles: A role for surface area and oxidative stress in the enhanced activity of ultrafines. *Toxicology and Applied Pharmacology*, 175(3), pp.191–199.

Carrillo, C., Suñé, J.M., Pérez-Lozano, P., García-Montoya, E., Sarrate, R., Fàbregas, A., Miñarro, M. and Ticó, J.R., 2014. Chitosan nanoparticles as non-viral gene delivery systems: Determination of loading efficiency. *Biomedicine and Pharmacotherapy*, 68(6), pp.775–783.

Chen, Q., Chen, J., Liang, C., Feng, L., Dong, Z., Song, X., Song, G. and Liu, Z., 2017. Drug-induced co-assembly of albumin/catalase as smart Nano-theranostics for deep intra-tumoral penetration, hypoxia relieve, and synergistic combination therapy. *Journal of Controlled Release*, 263, pp.79–89.

Couvreur, P., Dubernet, C. and Puisieux, F., 1995. Controlled drug delivery with nanoparticles: Current possibilities and future trends. *European Journal of Pharmaceutics and Biopharmaceutics*, 41(1), pp.2–13.

Dai, X., Yu, L., Zhang, Y., Zhang, L. and Tan, J., 2019. Polymerization-induced self-assembly via RAFT-mediated emulsion polymerization of methacrylic monomers. *Macromolecules*, 52(19), pp.7468–7476.

Davarpanah, E. and Guilhermino, L., 2019. Are gold nanoparticles and microplastics mixtures more toxic to the marine microalgae Tetraselmis chuii than the substances individually? *Ecotoxicology and Environmental Safety*, 181, pp.60–68.

De Campos, A.M., Diebold, Y., Carvalho, E.L., Sánchez, A. and José Alonso, M., 2004. Chitosan nanoparticles as new ocular drug delivery systems: in vitro stability, in vivo fate, and cellular toxicity. *Pharmaceutical research*, 21(5), pp.803–810.

DeLoid, G.M., Wang, Y., Kapronezai, K., Lorente, L.R., Zhang, R., Pyrgiotakis, G., Konduru, N.V., Ericsson, M., White, J.C., De La Torre-Roche, R., Xiao, H., McClements, D.J. and Demokritou, P., 2017. An integrated methodology for assessing the impact of food matrix and gastrointestinal effects on the biokinetics and cellular toxicity of ingested engineered nanomaterials. *Particle and Fibre Toxicology*, 14(1), pp.1–17.

Decuzzi, P., Godin, B., Tanaka, T., Lee, S.Y., Chiappini, C., Liu, X. and Ferrari, M., 2010. Size and shape effects in the biodistribution of intravascularly injected particles. *Journal of Controlled Release*, 141(3), pp.320–327.

Donaldson, K., Stone, V., Tran, C., Kreyling, W. and Borm, P.J., 2004. Nanotoxicology. *Occupational and Environmental Medicine*, 61(9), pp.727–728.

Fallah, Z., Zare, E.N., Ghomi, M., Ahmadijokani, F., Amini, M., Tajbakhsh, M., Arjmand, M., Sharma, G., Ali, H., Ahmad, A., Makvandi, P., Lichtfouse, E., Sillanpää, M. and Varma, R.S., 2021. Toxicity and remediation of pharmaceuticals and pesticides using metal oxides and carbon nanomaterials. *Chemosphere*, p.130055.

Fallah, A.A., Sarmast, E., Dehkordi, S.H., Isvand, A., Dini, H., Jafari, T., Soleimani, M. and Khaneghah, A.M., 2022. Low-dose gamma irradiation and pectin biodegradable nanocomposite coating containing curcumin nanoparticles and ajowan (Carum copticum) essential oil nanoemulsion for storage of chilled lamb loins. *Meat Science*, 184, p.108700.

Fard, J.K., Jafari, S. and Eghbal, M.A., 2015. A review of molecular mechanisms involved in toxicity of nanoparticles. *Advanced pharmaceutical bulletin*, 5(4), p.447.

Fattal, E., Rojas, J., Youssef, M., Couvreur, P. and Andremont, A., 1991. Liposome-entrapped ampicillin in the treatment of experimental murine listeriosis and salmonellosis. *Antimicrobial Agents and Chemotherapy*, 35(4), pp.770–772.

Ferji, K., Venturini, P., Cleymand, F., Chassenieux, C. and Six, J.L., 2018. In situ glyconanostructure formulation via photo-polymerization induced self-assembly. *Polymer Chemistry*, 9(21), pp.2868–2872.

Gallo, J., Holinka, M. and Moucha, C.S., 2014. Antibacterial surface treatment for orthopaedic implants. *International Journal of Molecular Sciences*, 15(8), pp.13849–13880.

Gallo, M.C., Pires, B.M., Toledo, K.C., Jannuzzi, S.A., Arruda, E.G., Formiga, A.L. and Bonacin, J.A., 2014. The use of modified electrodes by hybrid systems gold nanoparticles/Mn-porphyrin in electrochemical detection of cysteine. *Synthetic metals*, 198, pp.335–339.

Garnett, M.C. and Kallinteri, P., 2006. Nanomedicines and nanotoxicology: Some physiological principles. *Occupational Medicine*, 56(5), pp.307–311.

Goodman, C.M., McCusker, C.D., Yilmaz, T. and Rotello, V.M., 2004. Toxicity of gold nanoparticles functionalized with cationic and anionic side chains. *Bioconjugate Chemistry*, 15(4), pp.897–900.

Groneberg, D.A., Giersig, M., Welte, T. and Pison, U., 2006. Nanoparticle-based diagnosis and therapy. *Current Drug Targets*, 7(6), pp.643–648.

Gu, Z., Dang, T.T., Ma, M., Tang, B.C., Cheng, H., Jiang, S., Dong, Y., Zhang, Y. and Anderson, D.G., 2013. Glucose-responsive microgels integrated with enzyme nanocapsules for closed-loop insulin delivery. *ACS Nano*, 7(8), pp.6758–6766.

Guterres, S.S., Fessi, H., Barratt, G., Puisieux, F. and Devissaguet, J.P., 2000. Poly (rac-lactide) nanocapsules containing diclofenac: Protection against muscular damage in rats. *Journal of Biomaterials Science, Polymer Edition*, 11(12), pp.1347–1355.

Hagens, W.I., Oomen, A.G., de Jong, W.H., Cassee, F.R. and Sips, A.J., 2007. What do we (need to) know about the kinetic properties of nanoparticles in the body? *Regulatory Toxicology and Pharmacology*, 49(3), pp.217–229.

Haliullin, T.O., Zalyalov, R.R., Shvedova, A.A. and Tkachov, A.G., 2015. Hygienic evaluation of multilayer carbon nanotubes. *Meditsina Truda i Promyshlennaia Ekologiia*, 7(7), pp.37–42.

Hofmann-Amtenbrink, M., Grainger, D.W. and Hofmann, H., 2015. Nanoparticles in medicine: Current challenges facing inorganic nanoparticle toxicity assessments and standardizations. *Nanomedicine: Nanotechnology, Biology and Medicine*, 11(7), pp.1689–1694.

Iavicoli, I., Leso, V., Ricciardi, W., Hodson, L.L. and Hoover, M.D., 2014. Opportunities and challenges of nanotechnology in the green economy. *Environmental Health: A Global Access Science Source*, 13(1), pp.1–11.

Jahangiri, A. and Barghi, L., 2018. Polymeric nanoparticles: Review of synthesis methods and applications in drug delivery. *Journal of Advanced Chemical and Pharmaceutical Materials (JACPM)*, 1(2), pp.38–47.

Kallinteri, P., Higgins, S., Hutcheon, G.A., St. Pourçain, C.B. and Garnett, M.C., 2005. Novel functionalized biodegradable polymers for nanoparticle drug delivery systems. *Biomacromolecules*, 6(4), pp.1885–1894.

Kesharwani, P., Gajbhiye, V. and Jain, N.K., 2012. A review of nanocarriers for the delivery of small interfering RNA. *Biomaterials*, 33(29), pp.7138–7150.

Knight, C.G., 1981. *Liposomes, from Physical Structure to Therapeutic Applications*. North-Holland Biomedical Press ; Sole distributors for the U.S.A. and Canada, Elsevier North-Holland, Amsterdam, New York: Elsevier.

Kou, L., Bhutia, Y.D., Yao, Q., He, Z., Sun, J. and Ganapathy, V., 2018. Transporter-guided delivery of nanoparticles to improve drug permeation across cellular barriers and drug exposure to selective cell types. *Frontiers in Pharmacology*, 9, p.27.

Kumar, V., Sharma, N. and Maitra, S.S., 2017. In vitro and in vivo toxicity assessment of nanoparticles. *International Nano Letters*, 7(4), pp.243–256.

Kumari, A., Singla, R., Guliani, A. and Yadav, S.K., 2014. Nanoencapsulation for drug delivery. *Excli Journal*, 13, p.265.

Kümmerer, K., 2008. Pharmaceuticals in the environment–a brief summary. In: *Pharmaceuticals in the Environment* (pp. 3–21).Berlin, Heidelberg: Springer. https://doi.org/10.1007/978-3-540-74664-5_1.

La Spada, L. and Vegni, L., 2018. Electromagnetic nanoparticles for sensing and medical diagnostic applications. *Materials*, 11(4), p.603.

Landsiedel, R., Fabian, E., Ma-Hock, L., Wohlleben, W., Wiench, K., Oesch, F. and van Ravenzwaay, B., 2012. Toxico-/biokinetics of nanomaterials. *Archives of Toxicology*, 86(7), pp.1021–1060.

Lin, J., Li, Y., Li, Y., Wu, H., Yu, F., Zhou, S., Xie, L., Luo, F., Lin, C. and Hou, Z., 2015. Drug/dye-loaded, multifunctional PEG–chitosan–iron oxide nanocomposites for methotraxate synergistically self-targeted cancer therapy and dual model imaging. *ACS Applied Materials and Interfaces*, 7(22), pp.11908–11920.

Liu, Y., Xu, Y., Tian, Y., Chen, C., Wang, C. and Jiang, X., 2014. Functional nanomaterials can optimize the efficacy of vaccines. *Small*, 10(22), pp.4505–4520.

Love, S.A., Thompson, J.W. and Haynes, C.L., 2012. Development of screening assays for nanoparticle toxicity assessment in human blood: Preliminary studies with charged Au nanoparticles. *Nanomedicine*, 7(9), pp.1355–1364.

Lujan, H. and Sayes, C.M., 2017. Cytotoxicological pathways induced after nanoparticle exposure: Studies of oxidative stress at the 'Nano–bio'interface. *Toxicology Research*, 6(5), pp.580–594.

Luther, M., Brandner, J.J., Kiwi-Minsker, L., Renken, A. and Schubert, K., 2008. Forced periodic temperature cycling of chemical reactions in microstructure devices. *Chemical engineering science*, 63(20), pp.4955–4961.

Luther, W., Nass, R., Schuster, F., Kallio, M. and Lintunen, P., 2004. *Industrial Application of Nanomaterials-changes and Risks: Technology Analysis Future Technologies Division, Germany.*

Ma, X., Gong, N., Zhong, L., Sun, J. and Liang, X.J., 2016. Future of nanotherapeutics: Targeting the cellular sub-organelles. *Biomaterials*, 97, pp.10–21.

Maiti, S., Fournier, I., Brar, S.K., Cledon, M. and Surampalli, R.Y., 2016. Nanomaterials in surface water and sediments: Fate and analytical challenges. *Journal of Hazardous, Toxic, and Radioactive Waste*, 20(1), p.B4014004.

Maksymowych, W.P., Blackburn, W.D., Tami, J.A. and Shanahan, W.R., 2002. A randomized, placebo controlled trial of an antisense oligodeoxynucleotide to intercellular adhesion molecule-1 in the treatment of severe rheumatoid arthritis. *The Journal of Rheumatology*, 29(3), pp.447–453.

Martinez-Martinez, M., Rodríguez-Berna, G., Gonzalez-Alvarez, I., Hernández, M.A.J., Corma, A., Bermejo, M., Merino, V. and Gonzalez-Alvarez, M., 2018. Ionic hydrogel based on chitosan cross-linked with 6-phosphogluconic trisodium salt as a drug delivery system. *Biomacromolecules*, 19(4), pp.1294–1304.

Medina, C., Santos-Martinez, M.J., Radomski, A., Corrigan, O.I. and Radomski, M.W., 2007. Nanoparticles: Pharmacological and toxicological significance. *British Journal of Pharmacology*, 150(5), pp.552–558.

Meng, F., Cheng, R., Deng, C. and Zhong, Z., 2012. Intracellular drug release nanosystems. *Materials Today*, 15(10), pp.436–442.

Misra, R., Acharya, S. and Sahoo, S.K., 2010. Cancer nanotechnology: Application of nanotechnology in cancer therapy. *Drug Discovery Today*, 15(19–20), pp.842–850.

Mitragotri, S., Lammers, T., Bae, Y.H., Schwendeman, S., De Smedt, S.C., Leroux, J.C., Peer, D., Kwon, I.C., Harashima, H., Kikuchi, A. and Oh, Y.K., 2017. Drug delivery research for the future: expanding the nano horizons and beyond. *Journal of controlled release*, 246, pp.183–184.

Moshed, A., Mohammad, A., Islam Sarkar, M.K. and Khaleque, M., 2017. The Application of nanotechnology in medical sciences: New horizon of treatment. *American Journal of Biomedical Sciences*, 9(1), pp.1–14.

Mu, W., Chu, Q., Liu, Y. and Zhang, N., 2020. A review on nano-based drug delivery system for cancer chemoimmunotherapy. *Nano-Micro Letters*, 12(1), pp.1–24.

Muhammad, Q., Jang, Y., Kang, S.H., Moon, J., Kim, W.J. and Park, H., 2020. Modulation of immune responses with nanoparticles and reduction of their immunotoxicity. *Biomaterials Science*, 8(6), pp.1490–1501.

Muul, L.M., Tuschong, L.M., Soenen, S.L., Jagadeesh, G.J., Ramsey, W.J., Long, Z., Carter, C.S., Garabedian, E.K., Alleyne, M., Brown, M., Bernstein, W., Schurman, S.H., Fleisher, T.A., Leitman, S.F., Dunbar, C.E., Blaese, R.M. and Candotti, F., 2003. Persistence and expression of the adenosine deaminase gene for 12 years and immune reaction to gene transfer components: Long-term results of the first clinical gene therapy trial. *Blood, The Journal of the American Society of Hematology*, 101(7), pp.2563–2569.

Myllynen, P.K., Loughran, M.J., Howard, C.V., Sormunen, R., Walsh, A.A. and Vähäkangas, K.H., 2008. Kinetics of gold nanoparticles in the human placenta. *Reproductive Toxicology*, 26(2), pp.130–137.

Ndlovu, N., Mayaya, T., Muitire, C. and Munyengwa, N., 2020. Nanotechnology applications in crop production and food systems. *International Journal of Plant Breeding and Crop Science*, 7(1), pp.624–634.

Oberdörster, G., 2000. Pulmonary effects of inhaled ultrafine particles. *International Archives of Occupational and Environmental Health*, 74(1), pp.1–8.

Orive, G., Hernandez, R.M., Gascon, A.R., Calafiore, R., Chang, T.M., De Vos, P., Hortelano, G., Hunkeler, D., Lacik, I., Shapiro, A.J. and Pedraz, J.L., 2003. Cell encapsulation: Promise and progress. *Nature Medicine*, 9(1), pp.104–107.

Ramamoorth, M. and Narvekar, A., 2015. Non viral vectors in gene therapy-an overview. *Journal of Clinical and Diagnostic Research*, 9(1), p.GE01.

Ramos, A.P., Cruz, M.A., Tovani, C.B. and Ciancaglini, P., 2017. Biomedical applications of nanotechnology. *Biophysical Reviews*, 9(2), pp.79–89.

Reis, C.P., Neufeld, R.J., Ribeiro, A.J. and Veiga, F., 2006. Nanoencapsulation I. Methods for preparation of drug-loaded polymeric nanoparticles. *Nanomedicine: Nanotechnology, Biology and Medicine*, 2(1), pp.8–21.

Ribeiro, A.J., 2017. Preparation of drug-loaded polymeric nanoparticles. In: *Nanomedicine in Cancer* (pp. 171–214). Jenny Stanford Publishing, United Square, Singapore.

Ribeiro, A.R., Leite, P.E., Falagan-Lotsch, P., Benetti, F., Micheletti, C., Budtz, H.C., Jacobsen, N.R., Lisboa-Filho, P.N., Rocha, L.A., Kühnel, D. and Hristozov, D., 2017. Challenges on the toxicological predictions of engineered nanoparticles. *NanoImpact*, 8, pp.59–72.

Saeedi, M., Eslamifar, M., Khezri, K. and Dizaj, S.M., 2019. Applications of nanotechnology in drug delivery to the central nervous system. *Biomedicine and Pharmacotherapy*, 111, pp.666–675.

Sahay, G., Alakhova, D.Y. and Kabanov, A.V., 2010. Endocytosis of nanomedicines. *Journal of Controlled Release*, 145(3), pp.182–195.

Sajja, H.K., East, M.P., Mao, H., Wang, Y.A., Nie, S. and Yang, L., 2009. Development of multifunctional nanoparticles for targeted drug delivery and noninvasive imaging of therapeutic effect. *Current Drug Discovery Technologies*, 6(1), pp.43–51.

Sayes, C.M., Reed, K.L. and Warheit, D.B., 2007. Assessing toxicity of fine and nanoparticles: Comparing in vitro measurements to in vivo pulmonary toxicity profiles. *Toxicological Sciences*, 97(1), pp.163–180.

Senjen, R. (2013). Nanomedicine new solutions or new problems. *PhD, HCWH Europe*.

Shuhendler, A.J., Prasad, P., Chan, H.K.C., Gordijo, C.R., Soroushian, B., Kolios, M., Yu, K., O'Brien, P.J., Rauth, A.M. and Wu, X.Y., 2011. Hybrid quantum dot-fatty ester stealth nanoparticles: Toward clinically relevant in vivo optical imaging of deep tissue. *ACS Nano*, 5(3), pp.1958–1966.

Shuhendler, A.J., Prasad, P., Leung, M., Rauth, A.M., DaCosta, R.S. and Wu, X.Y., 2012. A novel solid lipid nanoparticle formulation for active targeting to tumor $\alpha(v)\beta(3)$ integrin receptors reveals cyclic RGD as a double-edged sword. *Advanced Healthcare Materials*, 1(5), pp.600–608.

Smith, D.J., Leal, L.G., Mitragotri, S. and Shell, M.S., 2018. Nanoparticle transport across model cellular membranes: When do solubility-diffusion models break down?. *Journal of Physics D: Applied Physics*, 51(29), p.294004.

Soares, S., Sousa, J., Pais, A. and Vitorino, C., 2018. Nanomedicine: Principles, properties, and regulatory issues. *Frontiers in Chemistry*, 6, p.360.

Stylianopoulos, T. and Jain, R.K., 2015. Design considerations for nanotherapeutics in oncology. *Nanomedicine: Nanotechnology, Biology and Medicine*, 11(8), pp.1893–1907.

Tinkle, S., McNeil, S.E., Mühlebach, S., Bawa, R., Borchard, G., Barenholz, Y., Tamarkin, L. and Desai, N., 2014. Nanomedicines: Addressing the scientific and regulatory gap. *Annals of the New York Academy of Sciences*, 1313(1), pp.35–56.

Vallet-Regi, M. and Tamanoi, F., 2018. Overview of studies regarding mesoporous silica nanomaterials and their biomedical application. *The Enzymes*, 43, pp.1–10.

Vega-Villa, K.R., Takemoto, J.K., Yáñez, J.A., Remsberg, C.M., Forrest, M.L. and Davies, N.M., 2008. Clinical toxicities of nanocarrier systems. *Advanced Drug Delivery Reviews*, 60(8), pp.929–938.

Viseras, C., Aguzzi, C., Cerezo, P. and Bedmar, M.C., 2008. Biopolymer–clay nanocomposites for controlled drug delivery. *Materials Science and Technology*, 24(9), pp.1020–1026.

Weeraman, C., Yatawara, A.K., Bordenyuk, A.N. and Benderskii, A.V., 2006. Effect of nanoscale geometry on molecular conformation: Vibrational sum-frequency generation of alkanethiols on gold nanoparticles. *Journal of the American Chemical Society*, 128(44), pp.14244–14245.

Whelan, J., 2001. Nanocapsules for controlled drug delivery. *Drug Discovery Today*, 23(6), pp.1183–1184.

Wierzbicki, M., Sawosz, E., Grodzik, M., Hotowy, A., Prasek, M., Jaworski, S., Sawosz, F. and Chwalibog, A., 2013. Carbon nanoparticles downregulate expression of basic fibroblast growth factor in the heart during embryogenesis. *International Journal of Nanomedicine*, 8, p.3427.

Xia, T., Kovochich, M., Liong, M., Madler, L., Gilbert, B., Shi, H., Yeh, J.I., Zink, J.I. and Nel, A.E., 2008. Comparison of the mechanism of toxicity of zinc oxide and cerium oxide nanoparticles based on dissolution and oxidative stress properties. *ACS nano*, 2(10), pp.2121–2134.

Zhang, M., Hong, Y., Chen, W. and Wang, C., 2017. Polymers for DNA vaccine delivery. *ACS Biomaterials Science and Engineering*, 3(2), pp.108–125.

Zhao, F., Zhao, Y., Liu, Y., Chang, X., Chen, C. and Zhao, Y., 2011. Cellular uptake, intracellular trafficking, and cytotoxicity of nanomaterials. *Small*, 7(10), pp.1322–1337.

Zhao, J. and Castranova, V., 2011. Toxicology of nanomaterials used in nanomedicine. *Journal of Toxicology and Environmental Health, Part B*, 14(8), pp.593–632.

Zhao, Z., Zhou, Z., Bao, J., Wang, Z., Hu, J., Chi, X., Ni, K., Wang, R., Chen, X., Chen, Z. and Gao, J., 2013. Octapod iron oxide nanoparticles as high-performance T2 contrast agents for magnetic resonance imaging. *Nature communications*, 4(1), pp.1–7.

Zhang, R.X., Li, J., Zhang, T., Amini, M.A., He, C., Lu, B., Ahmed, T., Lip, H., Rauth, A.M. and Wu, X.Y., 2018. Importance of integrating nanotechnology with pharmacology and physiology for innovative drug delivery and therapy–an illustration with firsthand examples. *Acta Pharmacologica Sinica*, 39(5), pp.825–844.

Zindler, F., Glomstad, B., Altin, D., Liu, J., Jenssen, B.M. and Booth, A.M., 2016. Phenanthrene bioavailability and toxicity to Daphnia magna in the presence of carbon nanotubes with different physicochemical properties. *Environmental Science and Technology*, 50(22), pp.12446–12454.

Zuckerman, J.E., Choi, C.H.J., Han, H. and Davis, M.E., 2012. Polycation-siRNA nanoparticles can disassemble at the kidney glomerular basement membrane. *Proceedings of the National Academy of Sciences of the United States of America*, 109(8), pp.3137–3142.

Zygmanski, P., Liu, B., Tsiamas, P., Cifter, F., Petersheim, M., Hesser, J. and Sajo, E., 2013. Dependence of Monte Carlo microdosimetric computations on the simulation geometry of gold nanoparticles. *Physics in Medicine and Biology*, 58(22), p.7961.

6 Quantum Dots: Can It Be a Potential Antiviral Agent and Nano-Carrier Tool for Efficient Drug Delivery for Combatting Viral Infections?

Tabassum Khair Barbhuiya,
Nirupam Das, and Partha Palit

CONTENTS

DOI: 10.1201/9781003243175-6

6.1 INTRODUCTION

Viral infection has emerged as a global burden, with the significant outbreak of COVID-19. The highly contagious viral infections have given the flu-like symptoms and diseases associated with different viruses such as the H1N1 influenza virus, Ebola virus, Zika virus, severe acute respiratory syndrome coronavirus (SARS-CoV), H5N1 bird flu virus, Middle East respiratory syndrome coronavirus (MERS-CoV), and human immunodeficiency virus (HIV). Due to the contagious nature of the infections, rapid viral division and fast genetic mutations of the virus, eradication of viral infections has become the current global challenge. The current prevention and treatment approaches for viral diseases include a wide range of vaccines and antiviral drugs alone or in combination with monoclonal and polyclonal therapies, respectively (Łoczechin et al., 2019, Kotta et al., 2020, Szunerits et al., 2015). By taking adequate preventive measures, early diagnosis of viral infections and systematic cure with targeted therapeutic approaches, it is possible to combat the severe illness associated with viral diseases. It is necessary to improve antiviral treatment approaches by exploring alternate treatment strategies to meet global requirements.

The advancements in the field of nanotechnology over the past two decades have significantly contributed towards the development of the healthcare sector. The nanomedicine-based pharmaceuticals that utilize the concept of modern chemistry and material sciences are widely used for targeted drug delivery. This covers several delivery systems like nanoparticles, carbon nanotubes, fullerenes, quantum dots (QDs), dendrimers, liposomes, micelles, and drug-polymer conjugates. These are capable of significantly enhancing the therapeutic efficacy of the drugs while minimizing the adverse effects (Wang et al., 2013b, Nazarov et al., 2009). The small size of nanomedicines provides superior pharmacokinetics and pharmacodynamic advantages over conventional therapeutics (Chan, 2006).

Nanomaterials have recently emerged as efficient tools for viral therapeutics, diagnostics, and drug-delivery agents. The small size, large surface area, tuneable lipid-water solubility, and surface modifications of nanoscale materials have imparted additional advantages for targeted anti-therapy to modulate the viral infection cycle. The large surface area of these materials enables the attachment of multiple ligands, which in turn interferes with the multivalent viral attachment, thereby blocking its entry into the host cells (Łoczechin et al., 2019, Szunerits et al., 2015). Despite significant developments in the field of nanomedicines, the broad range of concepts and utilities of each sub-class for different categories of disease has not been explored properly. In this chapter, we will describe the fundamental concepts related to structural properties, synthesis, characterization, and applications of QD-based nanoparticles with respect to antiviral therapeutics, diagnostics, and delivery systems.

6.2 QUANTUM DOTS: DEFINITION, STRUCTURAL FEATURE, AND SPECIAL PROPERTIES

6.2.1 QUANTUM DOTS AND THEIR STRUCTURE

Quantum dots (QDs) are a class of semiconductor-based nanocrystals, with a size of up to a few nanometres (1–10 nm) having tightly confined electrons in a three-dimensional (3D) space. They are usually referred to as clusters of colloidal nanostructures or artificial atoms, having zero dimensions (0D). QDs are either made up of single-element materials (core-only), e.g. germanium or silicon, or from semi-conductors like CdSe, PbSe, PbS, and CdTe, which are considered core-shell systems (Murray et al., 1993, Pattantyus-Abraham et al., 2010, Sumanth Kumar et al., 2016). In the latter case, the core is shielded by a shell made of materials with a wider bandgap, thereby improving the fluorescent property and preventing the leaching of the native QDs. This makes core-shell systems more desirable for biological applications. The QDs possess two distinct structural features: a large surface area and physically confined electrons that distinguish them from other bulkier molecules (Wang et al., 2012).

6.2.2 Special Properties of QDs

Like every semiconductor material, QDs possess an intrinsic band gap between the low energy (valence band) and the high-energy (conduction band) state. The electrons get excited into the conduction band on absorbing energy from the incident light or some thermal source, leaving behind the hollow-valence band (hole). The excited electron interacts with a hole by forming a weak electrostatic interaction when the crystal size is less than its Bohr radius. This electron-hole pair is termed an "exciton." Therefore, every QD has an exciton with a Bohr radius, within which the electrons are confined physically, termed "quantum confinement" (Kumar et al., 2018).

The electronic "quantum confinement" of a QD makes the molecular properties of materials that are intermediate between bulk semiconductors and discrete molecules. Unlike other nanomaterials, they exhibit varying physicochemical, mechanical, optical, and electronic properties depending on their size and shape. Therefore, by appropriate tailoring of these variables, the QDs are explored in several fields of electronics like laser diodes, solar cells, transistors, LED, biomedical imaging, and quantum computing. Nowadays, QDs are widely used as diagnostic tools and for the targeted delivery of drugs for cancer and other diseases (Medintz et al., 2005, Michalet et al., 2005, Qi and Gao, 2008).

The QDs also have a unique property to display multiple electron generation (MEG) with the incidence of a single photon having energy doubles the bandgap of the material. The high-energy photon, when hitting the electron at its ground state, excites the electron, which utilizes the excess energy to excite another electron. In conventional metals or semiconductors, there is only a 1:1 ratio of an incident photon to the excited electron. This MEG property has been found in PbSe, PbS, and CdSe QDs (Kumar et al., 2018).

The typical carbon quantum dots (CQDs) used for antiviral therapy possess some physicochemical properties like absorbance, photoluminescence, and electroluminescence. The π-π^* transition of sp^2 hybridized carbon atoms and n-π^* transition associated with heteroatoms (N, S and P) are responsible for absorption peaks in the UV-visible region. The photoluminescence property is greatly dependent on the size and shape of the material, which controls the emission wavelength and intensity (Wang et al., 2019). When the excited electrons from the conduction band return to the ground state, they lose energy in the form of a high-energy photon causing luminescence to occur. The luminescence of QDs is size-dependent. The small particles have a larger bandgap, and this requires more energy to get excited hence the emitting of light of higher energy and thus, a shorter wavelength and vice versa. The small-sized QDs (radii 2–3 nm) emit shorter wavelengths of visible light (violet, indigo, blue, and green) whereas the larger QDs (5–6nm radii) emit light of greater wavelength (yellow, orange, and red) (Hong, 2019, Kumar et al., 2018).

6.3 SYNTHESIS OF QDS

The QDs are generally synthesized by two methods: top-down and bottom-up methods. In top-down approaches, a bulk semiconductor is generally thinned using techniques like electron/X-ray beam lithography, ion, or chemical implantation to achieve a QD with a small diameter. The geometry and size of the QDs are controlled to achieve the desired optoelectronic effects. The bottom-up approach involves different self-assembly techniques, which are broadly classified into the wet-chemical method and vapour-phase method (Bera et al., 2010). In this section we will briefly discuss each synthetic method involved in the top-down and bottom-up schemes. **Figure 6.1** represents a general synthetic approach used for QD synthesis as below.

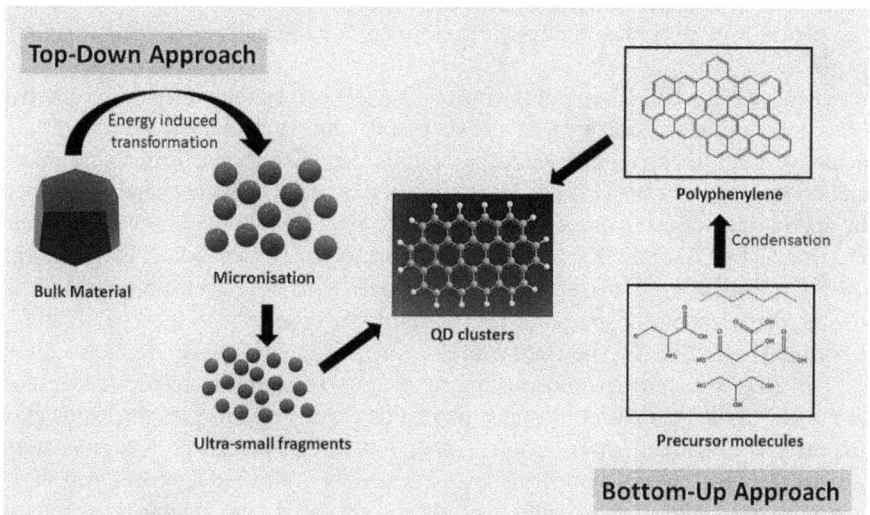

FIGURE 6.1 Representative scheme for top-down and bottom-up approaches for QD synthesis. In the top-down approach, the bulk material serving as the precursor gets micronized into ultra-small fragments by various physicochemical methods (electron beam lithography, reaction ion, and wet chemical etching, which are then fabricated to QDs. In the bottom-up approach, the precursor molecules are self-assembled by either wet chemical (sol-gel, microemulsion formation, hot-solution decomposition, and electrochemical) techniques or by the vapour-phase method (molecular beam epitaxy, sputtering, aggregations of gaseous monomers).

6.3.1   Top-Down Approaches

In the top-down process, the bulk of the precursor gets fragmented depending upon the size requirements. For example, electron beam lithography, reaction ion etching (RIE), and wet chemical etching are routinely utilized to get a QD of approximately 30 nm diameter. Laser beams or focused ions fabricate the array of zero-dimension (0D) QDs. But these methods incorporate structural imperfection due to patterning and impurities in QDs. The dry RIE etching involves the insertion of reactive gas into an etching chamber and a radio frequency voltage is applied to generate plasma that cleaves the gas molecules into more reactive species. These species with high kinetic energy strike the surface to form a volatile reaction product that etches a patterned sample.

The focused ion beam (FIB) technique utilizes focused beams from a molten metal source (e.g. Ga, Au/Si) to sputter the surface of the semiconductor substrate, and is also used to fabricate QDs with high precision. FIB can also selectively deposit a component from a precursor gas having resolution of approximately 100 nm. The use of electron beam lithography followed by etching or lift-off produces patterns with the required dimensions and possesses high flexibility for the design (Bera et al., 2010).

6.3.2   Bottom-Up Approaches

6.3.2.1   Wet-Chemical Methods

These methods involve self-assembly formation by the controlled precipitation of a single solution or mixtures by careful monitoring of critical process parameters and material attributes. The key parameters like concentration of precursor, temperature, the thickness of electrostatic double layer, type of stabilizers and solvents, and cationic-anionic species ratio are usually optimized to get an optimal QD of desirable shape and size. The sol-gel and microemulsion formation methods, hot-solution decomposition, and electrochemical techniques are a few that come under wet-chemical methods.

The sol-gel technique involves the formation of sol by dispersion (hydrolysis) of metal precursors like alkoxides, nitrates, or acetates in acidic/basic media, followed by polymerization into a gel, e.g. preparation of ZnO-QDs by mixing zinc acetate solution in alcohol and sodium hydroxide, followed by ariel growth (Bang et al., 2006). This is a simple, easily scalable, and cost-effective process. However, this method has limited use due to wide-ranging size distribution patterns and excessive concentration defects. The microemulsion (either oil-in-water or water-in-oil) method is widely used and involves preparing QDs at room temperature. The two immiscible liquids are vigorously stirred to form an emulsion in the presence of surfactants like Triton™-X, sodium dodecyl sulphate, and cetyl trimethyl ammonium bromide. This method is used to fabricate both single-core and core-shell QDs. The molar ratio of water to surfactant can be altered to control the size of QDs and this method gives narrow size distribution as compared to sol-gel. But with this method, a low yield is obtained and it is prone to include impurities and defects.

The high-solution decomposition process involves the dry mixing of metal-precursor (acetates, carbonates, oxides) and organometallic compound (tri-octyl phosphene selenide) and vigorous stirring at high temperature (~300°C) containing a dried coordinating solvent. This facilitates homogeneous nucleation for QDs and subsequent growth through the relatively slow Ostwald ripening process. The size and shape of QDs are generally controlled by the process parameters like reaction time, temperature, and material attributes like type and purity of solvents, coordinating agents, and the coordinating solvents. With this process, a large quantity of monodispersed and defect-free QDs can be synthesized which is usually compromised by the toxicity of some organometallic precursors, high production cost, and poor water solubility (Bera et al., 2010). In the other synthetic procedures, the electromagnetic waves (ultrasonic or microwaves) are passed through the mixtures of metal precursors in water, which assist their dissociation and the subsequent growth of QDs. Hydrothermal or other electrochemical synthesis involves crystallizing inorganic salts from water under low temperature and pressure. Monitoring the reaction time, temperature, pressure, etc. controls the size and shape of QDs (Bera et al., 2010).

6.3.2.2 Vapour-Phase Methods

The vapour-phase QD formation initiates with the layers grown at the atomic level leading to the formation of unpatterned self-assemblies. These self-assemblies are formed by methods like molecular beam epitaxy (MBE), and sputtering; aggregations of gaseous monomers are considered to be in this category. In MBE, the elemental, compound, or alloyed nanostructured components are deposited layer by layer as a thin film on a hot substrate that grows under an ultra-high vacuum. The beam in this process is formed from elements (e.g. As and Ga to make GaAs) or solid-gas combination (e.g. AsH_3, PH_3). The physical vapour deposition (PVD) yields layer growth by condensing vapours formed by thermal evaporation or sputtering into solids. Several other techniques can also facilitate evaporation, such as electron beam heating, Joule's heating, arc discharge, and pulsed laser ablation. Chemical vapour deposition (CVD) is an alternative way to obtain self-assembling QDs by forming a thin film. In this method, the precursors are allowed to diffuse to the heated substrate when placed in a chamber at a specific temperature and pressure. This leads to film formation and gaseous by-products, which desorb from the substrate when withdrawn from the chamber. Although these vapour-phase self-assembling methods provide template-independent QDs, the uneven size distribution causes heterogenous optoelectronic properties (Bera et al., 2010).

6.4 SURFACE MODIFICATION (FUNCTIONALIZATION) OF QDS

The various synthetic processes described in the previous section are carried out in high-temperature and organic solvents. In these synthetic methods, the surface of QD (both core and core-shell) is stabilized by hydrophobic ligands like amines or phosphenes as a measure to regulate the size and inhibit aggregations. This makes the structures inherently water insoluble. To be applicable in biological systems, either as delivery agents or biosensors, they must be aqueous soluble. Hence, different surface modification strategies to attach hydrophilic ligands, such as surface silanization, ligand exchange, and amphiphilic polymer coating are utilized to enhance solubility (Wang et al., 2012).

Surface silanization: This process involves coating QDs with a persistent layer of silica shell, which can crosslink with ligands, thereby forming a very stable capping. The process is initiated by exchanging surface ligands with thiol-containing silanes, e.g. mercaptopropyltris(methyloxy) silane (MPS). The trimethoxy silane (TMS) is then cross-linked with a siloxane bond. The final step involves the addition of modified silicon (aminopropyl silanes, PEG-silanes, phosphosilanes). The terminal groups at the silane shell expose their functional groups like thiol (-SH), phosphate (PO_4^{2-}), or alkyl group for further modifications (Karakoti et al., 2015, Wang et al., 2012).

Ligand exchange: This is the most common approach to stabilize the nanocrystals in an aqueous solution, where the native hydrophobic ligands viz. trioctylphosphine (TOP), trioctylphosphine oxide (TOPO), and hexadecyl amine (HDA) are exchanged with amphiphilic molecules having bifunctional groups at two ends (Thanh and Green, 2010). The thiols (–SH) functional groups are used as an anchor to attach to the surface of QDs, whereas the carboxyl (–COOH), amines (-NH₂), or hydroxyl (-OH) groups serve as the outer polar ends to improve solubility and further biomolecular attachment. The common bifunctional ligand exchange molecules such as cysteine, mercaptosuccinic acid, polyethylene glycol (PEG), mercaptoacetic acid (MAA), glutathione, polyamidoamine (PAMAM), and polyisoprene have greatly amplified the biomedical applications (Kairdolf et al., 2008, Thanh and Green, 2010, Karakoti et al., 2015).

Coating of amphiphilic polymers: In this method, the native hydrophobic surfactant layer (TOP/TOPO/HDA) on the QDs surface is retained. Instead, the QDs are coated with amphiphile, where the hydrophobic end of amphiphilic copolymers interacts with the hydrophobic surface of OD. The hydrophilic groups (carboxyl group or PEG chain) of block copolymer mediate the aqueous solubility and chemical modification. The cross-linking treatment during amphiphilic coating is considered to enhance the stability of the polymeric shell of QD (Karakoti et al., 2015, Wang et al., 2012).

The uncoated-bare QDs have high surface energies that bring about some surface defects, which have the capability to quench surface fluorescence. Moreover, uncoated QDs are susceptible to degradation by oxidative and photochemical reactions and their long-term exposure to biological fluid can leach the metal ions from the core, causing metal toxicity. To avoid surface defects and reactivity, the QDs are capped with agents, e.g., ZnS that enhance the stability and quantum yield.

The attachment of suitable functional groups is essential to anchor the biomolecules such as protein, DNA, peptides, and drug molecules on the QD surface for targeted therapy. The targeted delivery via bio-functionalization provides localized effects by enhancing the specificity towards the biological target and minimizing the off-target side effects. Two major attachment sites mediate the bio-functionalization: 1) the -SH bond between the sulphur groups of ZnS capped QDs and the amphiphilic thiol ligands/silanes and 2) hydrophobic interaction between the hydrophobic ligands of QDs and the end (hydrophobic) of amphiphilic copolymers such as poly(acrylic acid) and poly (maleic anhydride). The biomolecules can be attached by non-specific adsorption onto the large surface area of QDs, which generally depends on the electrostatic interaction with the biomolecules. The weak hydrogen bond interaction between biomolecules and ligands is also exploited to mediate the adsorption. The covalent coupling (amide or thiol) of functionally modified QDs with the free amino group or disulphide bond of protein, peptides and antibodies (Karakoti et al., 2015).

6.5   CHARACTERIZATION OF QDS

To characterize semiconductor QDs, it is essential to understand their composition, morphology, crystalline structure, optical properties, and the type of surface ligands. There are several thermal, microscopic, and spectroscopic techniques used for the qualitative and quantitative characterization of QDs. The representative diagram of the QD characterization techniques is illustrated in **Figure 6.2.**

Transmission electron microscopic (TEM) imaging provides an important platform for the determination of the size and distribution, and shape of the nanoparticles. It is easier to identify the surface morphology of QDs by TEM which is otherwise difficult to inspect by the visual identification method, wherein the size difference can be identified by a change in colour (in the case of CdSe QD) or by the infrared (IR) spectroscopy due to absorbance at the near-IR region (Moreels et al., 2009,

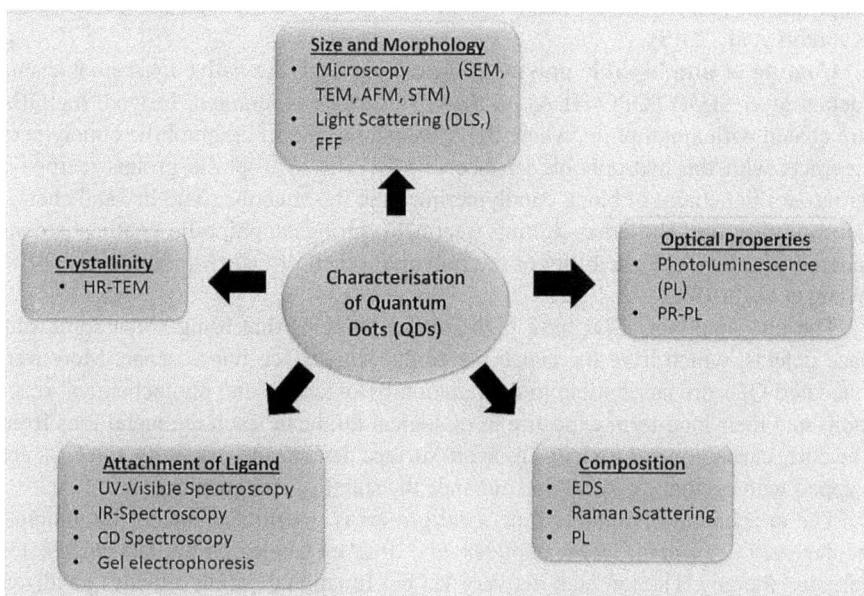

FIGURE 6.2   Methods for characterization (size and morphology, optical properties, composition, attachment of ligands and crystallinity) of quantum dots using various techniques.

Nordell et al., 2005). Other conventional size measurement methods are also used to characterize the size of QDs e.g. scanning electron microscopy (SEM) and dynamic light scattering (DLS). The optically active QDs made up of CdZnSe/ZnBeSe are characterized by their composition and size using a combination of techniques like photoluminescence, photoluminescence excitation, and Raman spectroscopy (Gu et al., 2003). Another group used the field flow fractionation (FFF) technique as a complementary tool to characterize the size of water-soluble CdSe-DNA-conjugated QDs (Rameshwar et al., 2006). The size of QDs prepared epitaxially, e.g. InGaN, InAs, and InGaAs can be monitored using atomic force microscopy (AFM) and scanning tunnelling microscopy (STM) (Hapke-Wurst et al., 1999, Yamauchi et al., 2001, Zhu et al., 2012). The qualitative analysis of the chemical composition of QDs can be done by energy dispersive spectrometry (EDS), Raman Scattering, and photoluminescence (PL) (Moreels et al., 2009).

The optical characteristic (fluorescence) of QDs can be determined by a variety of contactless, fast, and non-destructive techniques like photoluminescence (PL) and UV-visible spectroscopy. Another spectroscopic method, photo modulated reflectance (PR) spectroscopy in combination with PL has been explored to characterize the wetting layer and spacer analysis of low luminescence intensity QD structure stacked vertically (Drbohlavova et al., 2009, Hazdra et al., 2008). The high-resolution TEM (HRTEM) determines the crystallinity of QDs, impacting their thermal stability. Moreels et al. have developed the following semiempirical equation (1) to determine the energy band gap and optical properties, that utilizes the size measurements obtained from TEM analysis (Moreels et al., 2009, Pan et al., 2015):

$$E_0 = 0 \cdot 41 + \frac{1}{0.0252d^2 + 0 \cdot 283d} \tag{1}$$

Where, E_0 denotes the energy band gap (in eV), and d implies the diameter of QD (in nm).

The surface modification or functionalization of QDs by attaching various ligands expands its application in a wide range of areas. Hence it is essential to characterize the attached ligand. FT-IR spectroscopy enables us to understand the surface changes of the samples by identification of the IR bands corresponding to the stretching and bending energies of the functional groups attached (Pan et al., 2015). The bio-conjugated quantum dots e.g. the aptamer-functionalized can be characterized by UV-visible spectroscopy by analyzing the absorbance peak of the functional group of the conjugate. Gel electrophoresis (GE) is another technique that is widely used to characterize bio-conjugated systems. The main difference between the GE of QD-bioconjugate and other nano-bioconjugate is that the staining process is not used in the former case due to its inherent fluorescent characteristics. The circular dichroism (CD) spectroscopy measuring the ellipticity of optically active materials e.g. protein or oligonucleotides on interaction with circularly polarized light is generally used to determine the secondary structure of biomolecules. This technique also finds application in the characterization of QDs functionally modified with biomolecules like aptamer conjugated QDs (Yüce and Kurt, 2017).

6.6 CARBON-BASED QUANTUM DOTS AS NANOTHERAPEUTICS IN VIRAL DISEASES

In the last decade, carbon quantum dots have started to hold promise for delivering several antiviral agents, derived from natural, generic molecules to the host cell receptor. It was achieved due to the conjugation of host cell receptor-meditated specific ligands into the functionalized surfaces of carbon dots. As a result, surface-modified functionalized carbon dots can act as an effective drug delivery tool to get optimized antiviral response with minimized side effects. It also reduces the loading and frequency of doses of conventional and potent antiviral agents. This emerging and attractive drug carrier can formulate the potential drug in a safe, rapid and eco-friendly manner for improved drug delivery. The fabrication of carbon dots is carried out with the utilization of biodegradable, biocompatible, and cost-effective polymers via surface functionalization, for which it can safely deliver the active medicament to the locus of action as a potential self-made nano-carrier therapeutic carrier (Bawarski et al., 2008, Cohen et al., 2020). This technology involves nanoscience as well as quantum science, by which antiviral active medicament can be targeted to the culprit virus in a controlled released manner.

6.6.1 MECHANISM OF ACTION OF ANTIVIRAL QDs

Earlier literature entails that the antiviral mechanism elicited by active ingredient attached quantum dots includes the interference of four main steps viz. attachment, infiltration, replication, and budding in host cells. As attachment is a very important stage of viral infection to the host cells, inhibition of the attachment between viral surface protein and host cell surface receptor can significantly downregulate the further viral growth and infectivity into the host cells. Thus, it inactivates the virion infectivity by altering the viral surface protein. Several reports suggested that carbon dots can interact with the virus surface membrane protein to stabilize them for blocking their entry into host cells as evident from a study conducted by Huang et al., 2019 with carbon dots fabricated from benzoxazine monomeric units. It shows the entry inhibition of potentially fatal flaviviruses (Japanese encephalitis, Zika, and dengue) and naked viruses (parvovirus of porcine origin and adenovirus-associated virus) into host cells attaching surface receptors with significant IC_{50} (Huang et al., 2019). Moreover, Barras et al., 2016 demonstrate that carbon nanodots with a boronic acid or amine-functionalized surface interfere with the early steps of interaction of HSV-1 with the host cells resulting in the prevention of progressive infection. Carbon nanodots can act on the second stages of the virus life cycle once it prevents the infiltration of infective viral particles into host cells. These episodes involve the modification of the host cell surface attached membrane protein or direct blockage of the host cell surface receptor protein (Barras et al., 2016). As supported by Raman spectral and fluorescence analysis, the curcumin nano-carbon dots can stop the infection in the initial phase of viral entry. The study reported that positively charged carbon dots inactivates the virus via aggregation caused by electrostatic interaction of the nano-curcumin dots (Ting et al., 2020). A most interesting report suggested that ethylenediamine/citric acid-derived CQDs elicited its antiviral action against the coronavirus via interacting with the HCoV-229E entry receptors on host cells through its postmodified boronic acid functional group of surface ligands. It significantly promotes the blockage of the entry of HCoV-229E virus into the host cell surface receptor (Łoczechin et al., 2019). Our extended literature study illustrates that amine or boronic acid functionalized carbon nanodots can hinder the entry of type 1 herpes simplex virus by possibly with the host cells (Barras et al., 2016). So, penetration of HSV-1 virus into the intracellular region of host cells can be blocked to prevent infection by these emerging strategies of nano-carbon dots.

After entering infective virus particles into host cells, the only strategy to combat the infection is to prevent viral replication. It involves the inhibition of virus replicating enzymes such as DNA or RNA-dependent polymerase, main protease etc. that augments the viral genome replication inside the host cells. Blue-fluorescent CDs demonstrated a remarkable decrease of pseudorabies virus replication after significant distribution following entry into host cells by stimulating the antiviral state (upregulation of IFN-gamma followed by ISGs gene) of host cells (PK-15 cells) as assessed by plaque assay (Liu et al., 2017). That upregulated ISG and cytotoxic IFN cytokines can kill the newly replicated virus particles to prevent the budding and their detachment from the host cells to control the progression of infection. Moreover, positively charged curcumin carbon dots triggered a substantial decline in the synthesis of RNA strands (negative) in the porcine epidemic diarrhoea virus. The Vero cells demonstrate decreased plaque numbers and viral titre compared to an empty carbon-dots control group. (Ting et al., 2020).

Another significant antiviral drug target is to interfere with and block the budding of newly formed viral particles from the host cells. This episode occurs after replication followed by the excision of a more virulent and newly mutated daughter virus. Inhibition of budding and detachment of daughter virus particles by nano-carbon dots can effectively control and manage the severity of viral infection. Curcumin-carbon dots-180 effectively inhibit the Enterovirus 71 (EV71)-induced eIF4G cleavage and phosphorylated p38 kinase, for which the end stage budding and release of the newly synthesized virus particle would be stopped (Lin et al., 2019). However, expanded research studies are desirable to investigate all the possible modes of antiviral action of carbon dots in deactivating/suppressing or killing the virus. All the mechanisms of antiviral response elicited by different quantum dots with their various profiles have been presented in **Table 6.1.**

6.6.2 Significance of QDs in Drug Targeting

A virus lifecycle's major episode occurs within the host cells beginning from the cell surface membrane receptors' mediated attachment. So, quantum dot-mediated antiviral therapy should be explored as a target-oriented drug delivery towards the locus of action, particularly in the intracellular penetration and binding with the host

TABLE 6.1

Description of Numerous Quantum Dot-based Drug Conjugates Including Their Synthesis Method, Size Profile, Mechanism of Action, and Efficacy Profiles against Viral Infection

Nature of quantum dots Carbon-/ZnO-/ZnS-/Cd-based drug conjugates' profile	Size	Synthesis method	Effective against which viral diseases	Mechanism of antiviral activity	Outcome /degree of protection	Reference
Carbon quantum dots derived from curcumin (Cur-CQDs)	Range from 5.9 to 20.2 nm	Simply by heating at 120, 150, 180, or 210 °C followed by centrifugation and dialysis	Enterovirus 71 (EV71)	➤ Attachment of the EV71 virus to the cell membrane of host cells ➤ EV71-induced ROS production in host cells ➤ translation of EV71- and EV71-induced eIF4G cleavage & phosphorylated p38 kinase	CC_{50} 452.2[µg mL towards host c EC_{50} 0.2[µg/ml] with Cur-CQDs-180 for inhibition of EV71 infection towards EV71 with SI- 2261 Cur-CQDs-180 at a dose of 25 mg/kg body weight (bw) showed remarkable survival >95 after one month	Lin et al., 2019

(Continued)

TABLE 6.1 (CONTINUED)

Description of Numerous Quantum Dot-based Drug Conjugates Including Their Synthesis Method, Size Profile, Mechanism of Action, and Efficacy Profiles against Viral Infection

Nature of quantum dots Carbon-/ZnO-/ZnS-/Cd-based drug conjugates' profile	Size	Synthesis method	Effective against which viral diseases	Mechanism of antiviral activity	Outcome /degree of protection	Reference
Amino phenylboronic acid attributed carbon dots	Diameter size obtained by APBA-CDs -5 nm in HRTEM analysis	Amino phenylboronic acid-conjugated carbon dots were prepared from anhydrous citric acid (CA) and 2-amino phenylboronic acid (APBA) via pyrolysis via calcination on the isolated reactor at 270° for 4h and stable room temperature dissolving 1M NaOH solution Followed by neutralizing the solution using HCl.	Against AIDS virus	Block HIV-1 infection onto MOLT-4 cell via possible binding with gp120 protein of viral protein and boronic acid site of CDs to block the HIV and host cell interaction Delimitating of syncitia formation and higher ATP signal rather than bare carbon dots	EC_{50} 0.48 mg/ml Selectivity Index up to 3720.93	Aung et al., 2020

(*Continued*)

TABLE 6.1 (CONTINUED)

Description of Numerous Quantum Dot-based Drug Conjugates Including Their Synthesis Method, Size Profile, Mechanism of Action, and Efficacy Profiles against Viral Infection

Nature of quantum dots Carbon-/ZnO-/ZnS-/ Cd-based drug conjugates' profile	Size	Synthesis method	Effective against which viral diseases	Mechanism of antiviral activity	Outcome /degree of protection	Reference
Graphene quantum dots	5–10 nm with a round shape as per TEM and DLS analysis	Purified multi-walled carbon nanotubes obtained by catalytic chemical vapour deposition are subjected to oxidation under acidic oxidation ($HNO_3/H2SO_4$) for an extended period (4 days) by refluxing followed by sonication Coupling the $-NH_2$ groups of the anti-HIV drugs and -COOH functional groups of the nanotubes yielded the graphene quantum dots	Against HIV-induced AIDS	Inhibiting RNA-dependent DNA polymerase in vitro & reduction of HIV-1-induced cytopathic effect in MD4 host cells

A cleavable amide bond allows the release of the virus binding inhibitor GQD and the non-nucleoside reverse transcriptase inhibitor CHI499 | IC_{50} of 0.09 µg/MI RNA-dependent DNA polymerase and EC_{50} –0.066 µg/ mL HIV-1-induced cytopathic effect in MT-4 cells with SI- 362 by QGD-CHI499 | Iannazzo et al., 2018 |

(Continued)

TABLE 6.1 (CONTINUED)
Description of Numerous Quantum Dot-based Drug Conjugates Including Their Synthesis Method, Size Profile, Mechanism of Action, and Efficacy Profiles against Viral Infection

Nature of quantum dots Carbon-/ZnO-/ZnS-/ Cd-based drug conjugates' profile	Size	Synthesis method	Effective against which viral diseases	Mechanism of antiviral activity	Outcome /degree of protection	Reference
Hydrophilic carbon quantum dots of carrageenan or pullulan	Mean particle size over 2.1 ± 0.6 nm	Through hydrolysis and followed by hydrothermal techniques and dialysis of 10 g/L biopolymer (carrageenan or pullulan) for nucleation in presence of 40G/L NaOH solution	against MERS coronavirus infection	Inhibiting the viral multiplication of MERS-CoV via stimulating the antiviral ISG and IFN-∞	2.5 µg/L of both pullulan and carrageenan-based CQDs exhibited viral inhibition with 44.3% and 59.5%	Wang et al., 2008
Inorganic CdSe/ZnS QDs	Mean particle size mean diameter of 23.1 nm	The organic phase was encapsulated by amphiphilic alginate to attain biocompatible water-soluble QDs via phase transfer and the formation of colloidal complexes of QD–virus through electrostatic repulsion force generated from both negatively charged virus and QDs was neutralized by various concentrations of cationic polybrene	Against Viral infection caused by dengue virus	Exhibiting the potency of QD–virus complexes as bioprobes for broadcasting antiviral agents, allo phycocyanin	BHK-21 cells were incubated for one hour with allophycocyanin purified and then infected with QD–virus complexes for 30 min showing weak intracellular fluorescence by the allophycocyanin at 125 ug/ml	Wang et al., 2008

(Continued)

TABLE 6.1 (CONTINUED)

Description of Numerous Quantum Dot-based Drug Conjugates Including Their Synthesis Method, Size Profile, Mechanism of Action, and Efficacy Profiles against Viral Infection

Nature of quantum dots Carbon-/ZnO-/ZnS-/Cd-based drug conjugates' profile	Size	Synthesis method	Effective against which viral diseases	Mechanism of antiviral activity	Outcome /degree of protection	Reference
4-aminophenylboronic acid (4-APBA) based carbon quantum dots	9.2 ± 0.3 nm of best CQDs	Surface modification with hydrothermal carbonization with 4-aminophenylboronic acid hydrochloride	human coronavirus HCoV- 229E infections	Inhibition of the entry of HCoV via interaction between HCoV-229E entry receptors and functional groups of the CQDs	EC_{50} of 5.2 ± 0.7 µg/ml	Łoczechin et al., 2019
Carbon nanodots surface-functionalized with boronic acid or amine	96 nm for 4-AB/C-nanodots	4-aminophenylboronic acid hydrochloride (4-AB/C-dots) using a modified hydrothermal carbonization	Herpes simplex virus type 1 (HSV-1) infection	Block early step of the interaction of HSV-1 with the cell resulting in an inhibition of the infection	$EC_{50} = 80$ and 145 ng/ml on Vero and A549 cells, respectively	Barras et al., 2016
Benzoxazine monomer-derived carbon dots	BZM-CDs of 4.4 ± 0.6 nm	By heating the solution of benzoxazine monomer and NaOH aqueous solution in an autoclave at 180°C for 2 h. and followed by cooling, neutralization with HCL, centrifugation and finally dialysis of supernatant.	Life-threatening flaviviruses (such as Japanese encephalitis, Zika, and dengue viruses) and non-enveloped viruses (porcine parvovirus and adenovirus-associated virus)	obstructing the capacity of viruses to infect the host cells Via host-virus receptor-mediated interaction blockage	The EC_{50} of BZM-CDs : 18.63 µg ml-1 (JEV), 3.715 µg ml-1 (ZIKV), 37.49 µg ml-1 (DENV), 40.25 µg ml-1 (AAV), and 45.51 µg ml-1 (PPV)	Huang et al., 2019

(Continued)

TABLE 6.1 (CONTINUED)

Description of Numerous Quantum Dot-based Drug Conjugates Including Their Synthesis Method, Size Profile, Mechanism of Action, and Efficacy Profiles against Viral Infection

Nature of quantum dots Carbon-/ZnO-/ZnS-/Cd-based drug conjugates' profile	Size	Synthesis method	Effective against which viral diseases	Mechanism of antiviral activity	Outcome /degree of protection	Reference
2,2′-(ethylenedioxy) bis(ethylamine)-C-Dots and 3-ethoxypropylamine-C-Dots(EPA-C-Dots)	4–5nm in average diameter	Chemical functionalization of carbon nano-powders with 2,2′-(ethylenedioxy) bis(ethylamine) or 3-ethoxypropylamine	Human norovirus virus-like-particles (VLPs)	Binding to the surface of VLPs and followed by blocking of interaction between the active sites on the VLPs with the HBGA receptors	5 μg/mL EDA-C-Dots display 100% inhibition in GII.4 VLP bindings to the type A HBGA receptors	Dong et al., 2017

cell receptor for better management of the virus infection. Intracellular delivery of an antiviral drug can be delivered to the intracellular parts of host cells for targeted and pH-responsive drug delivery platform with ZnO-QDs as supported by earlier reports (Muhammad et al., 2011). Furthermore, fluorescent labels for cellular labelling, and intracellular sensors tagging in the drug-loaded quantum dots may improve the delivery efficiency in the intracellular region of the host cell, where viral replication occurs. This will finally require the QDs to undertake targeted intracellular as well as extracellular delivery, not only to specific cells but also to various subcellular organelles and compartments (Delehanty et al., 2009). Improved drug delivery through quantum dots can be achieved by optimizing the QD size, methods for QD biofunctionalization, and surface coating.

Luminescent semiconductor quantum dots (QDs) are a booming tool for efficient antiviral drug delivery towards the locus of action by conjugating with nanoscale fluorophore sensors. In order to understand the mechanisms of QDs mediated targeted drug delivery, researchers incorporated the rhodamine fluorescent agents, viral antigen-specific antibody, peptide or DNA aptamer, by which it can escape the endosomes to reach the cytosol and execute the antiviral action (Breger et al., 2015).

6.6.3   SAFETY ISSUES OF QUANTUM DOT-BASED THERAPEUTICS

A study revealed that photoluminescent carbon dots exhibited no substantial abnormality in the organs of the animals as assessed by acute, subacute, and genotoxicity studies (Wang et al., 2013a). Earlier investigations suggested that neutral carbon dots are safer without inducing any cellular abnormalities. However, negatively and positively charged carbon dots may elicit oxidative stress and cytotoxicity, respectively (Emam et al., 2017, Havrdova et al., 2016). However, poor stability may limit the long-term application of nanosized carbon dot-based nanomedicine (Mishra et al., 2018). Recently, European medical associations have formed an expert group on the investigation and fixing of regulatory issues associated with nano-carbon-dot-based medicine. The implementation of safety and design perceptions is necessary to anticipate the assessment of associated risk, alleviation, and uncertainties concerning health, including the protection of the environment in the initial stages of nanotechnological-based development of products, including carbon dots (Schmutz et al., 2020).

6.7   APPLICATION OF QDS

Quantum science-based nano-carbon dots are emerging as a drug carrier tool, diagnostic probe, bio-imaging, and theragnostic agent as reported by recent research studies. It is utilized as a commanding fluorescent probe for the quantitative detection and imaging of the diseased organ with long-term execution in a multiplexed manner via its optical property. The integrated nanostructure of quantum dots with their fluorescent probe-derived emitting detectable signal assists to identify, bind, and treat diseased cells. Therefore, the investigation and study of quantum dots are now an interesting subject due to their cohesive targeting, imaging, and therapeutic functionalities. Carbon quantum dots are also an excellent platform for delivering hydrophilic therapeutic armaments, viz. small interfering RNA and antisense oligodeoxynucleotide, peptides, antibodies, and aptamers. The designing approach involves immobilization by covalent or noncovalent interaction at the hydrophilic site of an amphiphilic polymer. Conjugation with organic fluorophores in carbon quantum dots may help to provide an innate signal for an extended duration and real-time imaging of drug transport within the in-vivo system with selective drug delivery. A recent report of novel manganese carbon quantum dots (Mn/CQD/SiO2) with a non-invasive and biocompatible nano-carrier having a simplistic design displayed excellent biodistribution and proper delivery of the painkiller naproxen to the locus of action (Ardestani et al., 2021). This approach is clear evidence in support of the above concept in experiments. Another example illustrated that biofunctionalized carbon quantum dots conjugated with fluorescent nanomaterials and reactive target-specific functional groups can act for the dual action of targeted imaging and drug delivery (Kundu et al., 2021). Thus, surface-functionalized quantum dots with selective ligands or fluorescent probes will offer valuable information in the rational design of drug carriers that are biocompatible, potential agents for in-vivo drug screening, as well as an alternative validation tool for drug research (Jin et al., 2011, Qi and Gao, 2008).

6.7.1 ROLE OF ZNO-/ZNS-/CD-BASED QDs ON THE ANTIVIRAL ACTIVITY AND DRUG DELIVERY

The aqueous dispersion of CdTe/CdS/ZnS Core-Shell-based carbon nanodots, prepared by microwave synthesis, hold prolonged biocompatibility and photostability. This type of nano-carbon dot displays interesting inhibition on NF-κB signalling, for which a promising anti-inflammatory response is achieved during the viral replication. This is because CdTe QDs significantly stop the HSV-1-induced NF-kB activation and reduce the viral replication rate without activating AKT, and the ERK signalling pathways (Hu et al., 2016). This observation may imply that Cd-based quantum dots can control the unregulated cytokine storm-induced inflammatory response against unprecedented viral replication. Host cell surface receptor-specific targeting and well-predicted controlled drug delivery at the target site could be achieved with the quantum dots composed of numerous colloidal core/shell CdTe/CdSe, CdSe/ZnS, and InP/ZnS. It can deliver an antiviral agent very nicely at the target site as proven by earlier reports of anti-cancer drug delivery (Mathew et al., 2010).

6.7.2 ROLE OF QD-BASED 3D NANO-PRINTING ON ANTIVIRAL DRUG DELIVERY

The introduction of advanced 3-D printing technology into carbon nanodots gives an emerging dimension for antiviral drug delivery and virus detection. For the quantum dot as a model active drug-delivery tool, the potential antiviral agents can be coated by 3-D inkjet printing techniques to form a stereolithography-based polymer-coated microneedle for transdermal drug delivery (Boehm et al., 2011, 2014, 2013, 2012). Principally, this method could be convenient for superficial therapy of herpes simplex viral infection. The microneedles coated with quantum dots and antiviral agents may elicit some functionalized changes to the microneedle external surface and geometry, accredited to the wetting of the microneedle surface by 3-D nano-printing. Thus, quantum dot-based 3-D nano-printing can act as a promising theragnostic tool.

6.8 CONCLUSION

Our above-mentioned compiled study infers that antiviral or fluorochrome-doped carbon nanodots have played a significant role in fundamental pharmacology, especially in disease diagnostics, therapy, and non-hazardous user-friendly drug delivery. Taking a cue from the exclusive surface property and structural modification feasibility such as adjustable nano size, unique active medicament tagging, and doping mechanism, broad-spectrum surface-functionalized reactive groups have authorized an emerging opportunity for investigations, including viz. controlled, predictable, perceptible, and target delivery of QD-based drug formulations. It can be hypothesized that host cell surface receptor-mediated ligand tagging in carbon dots can minimize the intracellular toxicity of the nano-formulation. However, the chronic toxicity of some metal and organic fluorophore probe-tagged carbon nanodots is unidentified at present and needs to be examined thoroughly before in-vivo evaluation. Despite this limitation, QDs have proved helpful in cell and pre-clinical studies as nano-carriers of drugs, remarkable drug screening/validation detection tools, and disease diagnosis. Designing QDs with safe carbon materials or masking the toxic materials from host tissue exposure followed by rapid clearance from the body may realize therapeutically safe QDs with viable clinical relevance. The significant challenges involved in well-predicted drug-delivery approaches are transferring the active drug particle towards the site of action at proper concentration and bypassing the unwanted side effect. To achieve this therapeutic mission, there needs to be a systematic investigation of the QDs. Putatively, bio-engineered QDs would stabilize and surge the time of circulation in the plasma while dropping the concentration of the free drug to reduce the adverse drug reaction and achieve the pre-determined controlled release of a drug. Additionally, the targeting of therapeutic medicament may be achieved by linking the drug to the QD surface functional groups via cleavable covalent bonds, thereby avoiding initial renal elimination of the bioconjugates. After that, the ligands undergo elimination by splitting into smaller entities. These brilliant multi-purpose with minimally toxic or non-toxic nano-devices for drug therapy and delivery can be highlighted for future drug development tools subject to their in-depth pre-clinal and clinical validation. With developments focused on searching for new targeting ligands, particularly bio-active potential phytopharmaceuticals, the building of specialized surface-functionalized nanoparticles, and the implementation of the sophisticated principle of conjugation chemistry, the nanobiotechnological field is exploring the various excellent applications of QDs in the health care system.

REFERENCES

Ardestani, M. S., Zaheri, Z., Mohammadzadeh, P., Bitarafan-Rajabi, A. & Ghoreishi, S. M. 2021. Novel manganese carbon quantum dots as a nano-probe: Facile synthesis, characterization and their application in naproxen delivery (Mn/CQD/SiO2@ naproxen). *Bioorganic Chemistry*, 115, 105211.

Aung, Y. Y., Kristanti, A. N., Khairunisa, S. Q., Nasronudin, N., & Fahmi, M. Z. 2020. Inactivation of HIV-1 infection through integrative blocking with amino phenylboronic acid attributed carbon dots. *ACS Biomaterials Science & Engineering*, 6(8), 4490–4501.

Bang, J., Yang, H. & Holloway, P. H. 2006. Enhanced and stable green emission of ZnO nanoparticles by surface segregation of Mg. *Nanotechnology*, 17(4), 973.

Barras, A., Pagneux, Q., Sane, F., Wang, Q., Boukherroub, R., Hober, D. & Szunerits, S. 2016. High efficiency of functional carbon nanodots as entry inhibitors of herpes simplex virus type 1. *ACS Applied Materials and Interfaces*, 8(14), 9004–9013.

Bawarski, W. E., Chidlowsky, E., Bharali, D. J. & Mousa, S. A. 2008. Emerging nanopharmaceuticals. *Nanomedicine*, 4(4), 273–282.

Bera, D., Qian, L., Tseng, T.-K. & Holloway, P. H. 2010. Quantum dots and their multimodal applications: A review. *Materials*, 3(4), 2260–2345.

Boehm, R., Miller, P., Hayes, S., Monteiro-Riviere, N. & Narayan, R. 2011. Modification of microneedles using inkjet printing. *AIP Advances*, 1(2), 022139.

Boehm, R. D., Miller, P. R., Daniels, J., Stafslien, S. & Narayan, R. J. 2014. Inkjet printing for pharmaceutical applications. *Materials Today*, 17(5), 247–252.

Boehm, R. D., Miller, P. R., Schell, W. A., Perfect, J. R. & Narayan, R. J. 2013. Inkjet printing of amphotericin B onto biodegradable microneedles using piezoelectric inkjet printing. *JOM*, 65(4), 525–533.

Boehm, R. D., Miller, P. R., Singh, R., Shah, A., Stafslien, S., Daniels, J. & Narayan, R. J. 2012. Indirect rapid prototyping of antibacterial acid anhydride copolymer microneedles. *Biofabrication*, 4(1), 011002.

Breger, J., Delehanty, J. B. & Medintz, I. L. 2015. Continuing progress toward controlled intracellular delivery of semiconductor quantum dots. *Wiley Interdisciplinary Reviews: Nanomedicine and Nanobiotechnology*, 7(2), 131–151.

Chan, V. S. 2006. Nanomedicine: An unresolved regulatory issue. *Regulatory Toxicology and Pharmacology*, 46(3), 218–224.

Cohen, E. N., Kondiah, P. P. D., Choonara, Y. E., Du Toit, L. C. & Pillay, V. 2020. Carbon dots as nanotherapeutics for biomedical application. *Current Pharmaceutical Design*, 26(19), 2207–2221.

Delehanty, J. B., Mattoussi, H. & Medintz, I. L. 2009. Delivering quantum dots into cells: Strategies, progress and remaining issues. *Analytical and Bioanalytical Chemistry*, 393(4), 1091–1105.

Dong, X., Moyer, M. M., Yang, F., Sun, Y.-P., & Yang, L. 2017. Carbon dots' antiviral functions against noroviruses. *Scientific Reports*, 7(1), 1–10.

Drbohlavova, J., Adam, V., Kizek, R. & Hubalek, J. 2009. Quantum dots—Characterization, preparation and usage in biological systems. *International Journal of Molecular Sciences*, 10(2), 656–673.

Emam, A., Loutfy, S. A., Mostafa, A. A., Awad, H. & Mohamed, M. B. 2017. Cyto-toxicity, biocompatibility and cellular response of carbon dots–plasmonic based nano-hybrids for bioimaging. *RSC Advances*, 7(38), 23502–23514.

Gu, Y., Kuskovsky, I. L., Fung, J., Robinson, R., Herman, I., Neumark, G., Zhou, X., Guo, S. & Tamargo, M. 2003. Determination of size and composition of optically active CdZnSe/ZnBeSe quantum dots. *Applied Physics Letters*, 83(18), 3779–3781.

Hapke-Wurst, I., Zeitler, U., Schumacher, H., Haug, R., Pierz, K. & Ahlers, F. 1999. Size determination of InAs quantum dots using magneto-tunnelling experiments. *Semiconductor
Science and Technology*, 14(11), L41.

Havrdova, M., Hola, K., Skopalik, J., Tomankova, K., Petr, M., Cepe, K., Polakova, K., Tucek,
J., Bourlinos, A. B. & Zboril, R. 2016. Toxicity of carbon dots–Effect of surface func-
tionalization on the cell viability, reactive oxygen species generation and cell cycle.
Carbon, 99, 238–248.

Hazdra, P., Voves, J., Oswald, J., Kuldová, K., Hospodková, A., Hulicius, E. & Pangrác, J.
2008. Optical characterisation of MOVPE grown vertically correlated InAs/GaAs
quantum dots. *Microelectronics Journal*, 39(8), 1070–1074.

Hong, N. H. 2019. Introduction to nanomaterials: Basic properties, synthesis, and characterization. In *Micro and Nano Technologies, Nano-Sized Multifunctional Materials.*
Hong, N. H. (ed.). Oxford, United Kingdom: Elsevier, pp. 1–19.

Hu, Z., Song, B., Xu, L., Zhong, Y., Peng, F., Ji, X., Zhu, F., Yang, C., Zhou, J., Su, Y., Chen,
S., He, Y. & He, S. 2016. Aqueous synthesized quantum dots interfere with the NF-κB
pathway and confer anti-tumor, anti-viral and anti-inflammatory effects. *Biomaterials*,
108, 187–196.

Huang, S., Gu, J., Ye, J., Fang, B., Wan, S., Wang, C., Ashraf, U., Li, Q., Wang, X., Shao,
L., Song, Y., Zheng, X., Cao, F. & Cao, S. 2019. Benzoxazine monomer derived car-
bon dots as a broad-spectrum agent to block viral infectivity. *Journal of Colloid and
Interface Science*, 542, 198–206.

Iannazzo, D., Pistone, A., Ferro, S., De Luca, L., Monforte, A. M., Romeo, R., Buemi, M. R.,
& Pannecouque, C. 2018. Graphene quantum dots based systems as HIV inhibitors.
Bioconjugate Chemistry, 29(9), 3084–3093.

Jin, S., Hu, Y., Gu, Z., Liu, L. & Wu, H.-C. 2011. Application of quantum dots in biological
imaging. *Journal of Nanomaterials*, 2011 https://doi.org/10.1155/2011/834139.

Kairdolf, B. A., Mancini, M. C., Smith, A. M. & Nie, S. 2008. Minimizing nonspecific cellular binding of quantum dots with hydroxyl-derivatized surface coatings. *Analytical
Chemistry*, 80(8), 3029–3034.

Karakoti, A. S., Shukla, R., Shanker, R. & Singh, S. 2015. Surface functionalization of quantum dots for biological applications. *Advances in Colloid and Interface Science*, 215,
28–45.

Kotta, S., Aldawsari, H. M., Badr-Eldin, S. M., Alhakamy, N. A., Md, S., Nair, A. B. & Deb,
P. K. 2020. Exploring the potential of carbon dots to combat COVID-19. *Frontiers in
Molecular Biosciences*, 7, 428.

Kumar, D. S., Kumar, B. J. & Mahesh, H. 2018. Quantum nanostructures (QDs): An overview.
In *Micro and Nano Technologies, Synthesis of Inorganic Nanomaterials*, Bhagyaraj,
S. M., Oluwafemi, O. S., Kalarikkal, N., & Thomas, S. (eds.). Woodhead Publishing
(Elsevier), Duxford, United Kingdom, 59–88.

Kundu, S., Ghosh, M. & Sarkar, N. 2021. State of the art and perspectives on the biofunctionalization of fluorescent metal nanoclusters and carbon quantum dots for targeted
imaging and drug delivery. *Langmuir*, 37(31), 9281–9301.

Lin, C. J., Chang, L., Chu, H. W., Lin, H. J., Chang, P. C., Wang, R. Y., Unnikrishnan,
B., Mao, J. Y., Chen, S. Y. & Huang, C. C. 2019. High amplification of the antiviral
activity of curcumin through transformation into carbon quantum dots. *Small*, 15(41),
1902641.

Liu, H., Bai, Y., Zhou, Y., Feng, C., Liu, L., Fang, L., Liang, J. & Xiao, S. 2017. Blue and cyan
fluorescent carbon dots: One-pot synthesis, selective cell imaging and their antiviral
activity. *RSC Advances*, 7(45), 28016–28023.

Łoczechin, A., Séron, K., Barras, A., Giovanelli, E., Belouzard, S., Chen, Y.-T., Metzler-Nolte,
N., Boukherroub, R., Dubuisson, J. & Szunerits, S. 2019. Functional carbon quantum

dots as medical countermeasures to human coronavirus. *ACS Applied Materials and Interfaces*, 11(46), 42964–42974.

Mathew, M. E., Mohan, J. C., Manzoor, K., Nair, S., Tamura, H. & Jayakumar, R. 2010. Folate conjugated carboxymethyl chitosan–manganese doped zinc sulphide nanoparticles for targeted drug delivery and imaging of cancer cells. *Carbohydrate Polymers*, 80(2), 442–448.

Medintz, I. L., Uyeda, H. T., Goldman, E. R. & Mattoussi, H. 2005. Quantum dot bioconjugates for imaging, labelling and sensing. *Nature Materials*, 4(6), 435–446.

Michalet, X., Pinaud, F., Bentolila, L., Tsay, J., Doose, S., Li, J., Sundaresan, G., Wu, A., Gambhir, S. & Weiss, S. 2005. Quantum dots for live cells, in vivo imaging, and diagnostics. *Science*, 307(5709), 538–544.

Mishra, V., Patil, A., Thakur, S. & Kesharwani, P. 2018. Carbon dots: Emerging theranostic nanoarchitectures. *Drug Discovery Today*, 23(6), 1219–1232.

Moreels, I., Lambert, K., Smeets, D., De Muynck, D., Nollet, T., Martins, J. C., Vanhaecke, F., Vantomme, A., Delerue, C., Allan, G. & Hens, Z. 2009. Size-dependent optical properties of colloidal PbS quantum dots. *ACS Nano*, 3(10), 3023–3030.

Muhammad, F., Guo, M., Guo, Y., Qi, W., Qu, F., Sun, F., Zhao, H. & Zhu, G. 2011. Acid degradable ZnO quantum dots as a platform for targeted delivery of an anticancer drug. *Journal of Materials Chemistry*, 21(35), 13406–13412.

Murray, C., Norris, D. J. & Bawendi, M. G. 1993. Synthesis and characterization of nearly monodisperse CdE (E= sulfur, selenium, tellurium) semiconductor nanocrystallites. *Journal of the American Chemical Society*, 115(19), 8706–8715.

Nazarov, G., Galan, S., Nazarova, E., Karkishchenko, N., Muradov, M. & Stepanov, V. 2009. Nanosized forms of drugs (a review). *Pharmaceutical Chemistry Journal*, 43(3), 163–170.

Nordell, K. J., Boatman, E. M. & Lisensky, G. C. 2005. A safer, easier, faster synthesis for CdSe quantum dot nanocrystals. *Journal of Chemical Education*, 82(11), 1697.

Pan, Y., Li, Y. R., Zhao, Y. & Akins, D. L. 2015. Synthesis and characterization of quantum dots: A case study using PbS. *Journal of Chemical Education*, 92(11), 1860–1865.

Pattantyus-Abraham, A. G., Kramer, I. J., Barkhouse, A. R., Wang, X., Konstantatos, G., Debnath, R., Levina, L., Raabe, I., Nazeeruddin, M. K., Gratzel, M. & Sargent, E. H. 2010. Depleted-heterojunction colloidal quantum dot solar cells. *ACS Nano*, 4(6), 3374–3380.

Qi, L. & Gao, X. 2008. Emerging application of quantum dots for drug delivery and therapy. *Expert Opinion on Drug Delivery*, 5(3), 263–267.

Rameshwar, T., Samal, S., Lee, S., Kim, S., Cho, J. & Kim, I. S. 2006. Determination of the size of water-soluble nanoparticles and quantum dots by field-flow fractionation. *Journal of Nanoscience and Nanotechnology*, 6(8), 2461–2467.

Schmutz, M., Borges, O., Jesus, S., Borchard, G., Perale, G., Zinn, M., Sips, Ä. A., Soeteman-Hernandez, L. G., Wick, P. & Som, C. 2020. A methodological safe-by-design approach for the development of nanomedicines. *Frontiers in Bioengineering and Biotechnology*, 8, 258.

Sumanth Kumar, D., Jai Kumar, B., & Mahesh, H. M. 2016. Optical properties of colloidal aqueous synthesized 3 mercaptopropionic acid stabilized CdS quantum dots. *American Institute of Physics Conference Series*,1728, 020162.

Szunerits, S., Barras, A., Khanal, M., Pagneux, Q. & Boukherroub, R. 2015. Nanostructures for the inhibition of viral infections. *Molecules*, 20(8), 14051–14081.

Thanh, N. T. & Green, L. A. 2010. Functionalisation of nanoparticles for biomedical applications. *Nano Today*, 5(3), 213–230.

Ting, D., Dong, N., Fang, L., Lu, J., Bi, J., Xiao, S. & Han, H. 2020. Correction to multisite inhibitors for enteric coronavirus: Antiviral cationic carbon dots based on curcumin. *ACS Applied Nano Materials*, 3(5), 4913–4913.

Wang, C.-H., Hsu, Y.-S., & Peng, C.-A. 2008. Quantum dots encapsulated with amphiphilic alginate as bioprobe for fast screening anti-dengue virus agents. *Biosensors and Bioelectronics*, 24(4), 1012–1019.

Wang, J., Han, S., Ke, D. & Wang, R. 2012. Semiconductor quantum dots surface modification for potential cancer diagnostic and therapeutic applications. *Journal of Nanomaterials*, 2012 https://doi.org/10.1155/2012/129041.

Wang, K., Gao, Z., Gao, G., Wo, Y., Wang, Y., Shen, G. & Cui, D. 2013a. Systematic safety evaluation on photoluminescent carbon dots. *Nanoscale Research Letters*, 8(1), 1–9.

Wang, R., Billone, P. S. & Mullett, W. M. 2013b. Nanomedicine in action: An overview of cancer nanomedicine on the market and in clinical trials. *Journal of Nanomaterials*, 2013 https://doi.org/10.1155/2013/629681.

Wang, X., Feng, Y., Dong, P. & Huang, J. 2019. A mini-review on carbon quantum dots: Preparation, properties, and electrocatalytic application. *Frontiers in Chemistry*, 7, 671.

Yamauchi, T., Matsuba, Y., Ohyama, Y., Tabuchi, M. & Nakamura, A. 2001. Quantum size effects of InAs-and InGaAs-quantum dots were studied by scanning tunnelling microscopy/spectroscopy. *Japanese Journal of Applied Physics*, 40, 2069.

Yüce, M. & Kurt, H. 2017. How to make nanobiosensors: Surface modification and characterisation of nanomaterials for biosensing applications. *RSC Advances*, 7(78), 49386–49403.

Zhu, T., El-Ella, H. A., Reid, B., Holmes, M. J., Taylor, R. A., Kappers, M. J. & Oliver, R. A. 2012. Growth and optical characterisation of multilayers of InGaN quantum dots. *Journal of Crystal Growth*, 338(1), 262–266.

7 Small Molecule Antivirals to Nanoparticles
The Need of the Hour to Combat Pandemics

Sara Jones, Karthika Suryaletha,
and Akhila Velappan Savithri

CONTENTS

DOI: 10.1201/9781003243175-7

7.1 INTRODUCTION

Infectious diseases are as old as human civilization, and disease caused by viruses always remains one of the prime concerns. Viruses consist of DNA or RNA as their genetic material and are obligate parasites, which means they need a host cell for viral replication. Several new viruses have caused significant outbreaks globally with pandemic potential in the past years. Several factors are responsible for the difficulty in developing a foolproof antiviral therapy against viral infections. Recent developments in understanding virus genetic, structural, and functional diversities, their replication, and their association with host immune responses have helped find specific targets for developing antiviral drugs against a few viruses. And with the advancement in the field of nanotechnology, researchers have focused on the benefits of nanocarriers for drug delivery for enhancing antiviral efficacy and thus contributing to the current disease treatment against emerging pandemics.

7.2 COMPREHENSIVE TIMELINE CHRONICLES OF VIRAL PANDEMICS

The human race is currently traversing through the wreaking havoc of Severe Acute Respiratory Syndrome Corona Virus 2 (SARS-CoV-2), which is presently considered the sixth significant public health emergency of global concern.[1] It has barely left any part of the world unchanged, triggering landslide challenges to health and socio-economic parameters globally. Yet, this is not the first pandemic faced by the international community. Since time immemorial, several pandemic outbreaks ranging from asymptomatic to lethal stemmed from emerging and existing microbes worldwide. Although these outbreaks have wiped out millions of human and animal lives, paradoxically, they flagged the way for innovations in science and technology.

The Spanish flu outbreak caused by the H1N1 strain of influenza virus occurred in the twentieth century and is generally considered the first true global pandemic. Even though uncertainties abound concerning the time the influenza virus began to infect humans, many agree that the first pandemic could have occurred in 1510 A.D. The Spanish flu had an immense impact on global civilization as it determined the outcome of World War I. The genetic reassortment between different circulating strains of the influenza virus created a critical challenge in the emergence of new flu pandemics, the Asian flu, Hong Kong flu, and swine flu. The last few decades have witnessed some fatal viral pandemics with significant repercussions for societies across the globe. The major pandemics comprised the Human Immunodeficiency Virus in 1981, the Severe Acute Respiratory Syndrome Coronavirus-1 in 2002, the Influenza A (H1N1) 2009 virus, the Middle East Respiratory Syndrome Coronavirus in 2021, the Ebola virus in 2013, the Zika virus in 2015, and the present Severe Acute Respiratory Syndrome Coronavirus-2 circulating from 2019 till date.[2] Climate and anthropogenic changes facilitate virus spillover into broad geographical areas, increasing pandemic risk.

Moreover, the WHO has prioritized and enlisted these diseases for immediate studies in emergency contexts.[1] Besides, this list also includes Disease X, a hypothetical illness with an unknown entity speculated to cause a pandemic in the future with devastating effects across continents.[3] Disease X is undoubtedly the SARS-CoV-2 outbreak persisting worldwide in the current scenario. Infectious disease outbreaks of viral origin prevail and constitute a substantial global health burden.

7.3 ANTIMICROBIALS: TOOLS TO TACKLE INFECTIOUS DISEASES

Antimicrobials are one of the most fruitful forms of chemotherapy critical for the prophylactic and therapeutic management of infections. The primeval evidence of successful antimicrobial chemotherapy is from ancient Peru and China, where people used the bark of cinchona trees to reduce malaria incidence and severity. Interestingly, many of the ancient poultices used by primitive people had significant antiviral and antibacterial agents. In 1910[4] the discovery of p-rosaniline, an antitrypanosomal drug, and arsphenamine, an anti-syphilis drug by Paul Ehrlich, are both considered milestones in modern chemotherapy. He postulated the "magic bullet" concept, conveying that certain chemicals can selectively act against parasites without harming humans. However, it had limited success until Gerhard Domagk discovered the antibacterial properties of prontosil in 1930.[5] Of note, in 1929, penicillin G was already discovered by Fleming. But the magnitude of his revolutionary discovery gained the limelight only after ten years when Florey and his colleagues isolated and identified its protective action.[6] The advancement in fermentation techniques and biochemistry fuelled the synthesis of many innovative antimicrobial agents, emphasizing antibacterial agents. However, the development of effective nontoxic antivirals and antifungals has been at a snail-like pace and limited to antibacterials.

7.4 DELINEATION OF ANTIVIRALS

The SARS-CoV-2 outbreak has exposed the requisite for a technical breakthrough in antiviral therapy to curb the current crisis and curtail future attacks caused by other viruses of an unknown entity. Indeed, prevention by vaccination and treatment using antivirals/antibodies is the universally accepted keystone strategy followed in combatting viral diseases. However, the time required to develop a successful vaccine against any infectious disease is usually between five to ten years or longer. Also, there are occasions when vaccination is insufficient to improve the viral load, necessitating the development of antiviral agents. Currently, only 50 clinically approved antiviral drugs are available, and these are used explicitly against ten of the 220 viruses known to infect humans (Adamson et al., 2021).[7] Figure 7.1 demonstrates the discovery of significant antivirals throughout history. In 1963, idoxuridine, developed as an anticancer drug, became the first Food and Drug Administration (FDA) approved antiviral drug.

Antiviral therapies demand a better understanding of the structure of individual viruses and their specific interaction with host cells. Each virus has a unique structure, and they periodically alter the composition of the antigenic proteins, which are crucial in eliciting immune responses in the body. Since the virus depends on the host cell for its surveillance and replication, the antiviral agent must retard the virus infectivity without damaging the host cells. Various organic compounds, small

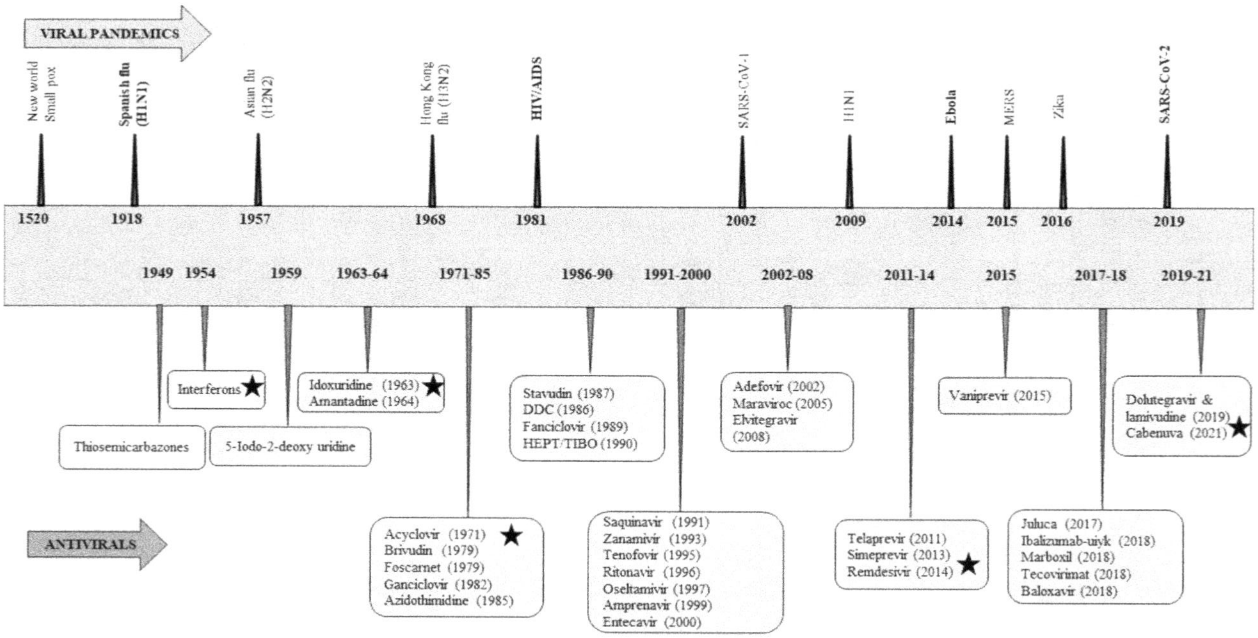

FIGURE 7.1 History of viral pandemics and the successive development of antiviral agents. Bold-Pandemics that instigated devastating effects across the globe. ★ Depicts the development of major antivirals which act as a breakthrough in antiviral treatment.

organic molecules, and biologics exert antiviral activity, but many responses were observed against the therapeutic management of different viruses. The development of antiviral resistance is the major stumbling block in the evolution of these agents, especially in RNA viruses, due to the error-prone nature of RNA-dependent RNA polymerase.[8] Hence, judicious use of these chemotherapeutic agents should be encouraged and newer strategies adopted to develop specific antiviral agents.

7.5 CLASSIFICATION OF ANTIVIRALS: SEQUELAE OF THE MODE OF ACTION

The strategies used to classify antiviral drugs are complex and interdependent. Antiviral agents are broadly classified based on their targets, mechanism of action, and chemical structures. Of note, many of the antiviral agents target either viral surface proteins or viral enzymes to prevent their entry and replication inside the host, as shown in Figure 7.2. The initial event in viral infection is the binding of the virus to the specific attachment sites widely distributed over the host cell membrane. Attachment inhibitors block viral interaction by targeting either viral surface proteins or cell surface receptors (Fostemsavir tromethamine, BMS-488043, BMS-663068). After attaching to host cell receptors, viruses use either endocytic or non-endocytic routes to enter the cell, releasing the viral genetic material into the host cytoplasm. Hence entry inhibitors play a crucial role in antiviral therapies by blocking the conformational changes required for membrane fusion. T20 (Enfuvirtide), the first and the only FDA-approved fusion inhibitor, is found to inhibit a broad range of enveloped viruses, especially HIV-1.[9] Enfuvirtide prevents the entry of HIV by inhibiting final fusion and thus protecting against further infection. Pleconaril, an entry inhibitor, prevents human rhinovirus from attaching to the host cell. Once inside the host cell, viral genomic nucleic acid, either DNA or RNA, is released by uncoating the viral capsid via enzyme degradation or dissociation.[10] Amantadine and rimantadine are good examples of uncoating inhibitors of the influenza A virus by preventing the virus release.[11–15] Once the virus enters the cell, virus replication and translation occur, resulting in viral protein components. The use of remdesivir, in case of SARS-CoV-2 and ribavirin, in case of respiratory syncytial virus and hepatitis C virus, which are nucleoside analogs, functions by blocking RNA-dependent RNA polymerase (RdRp) during mRNA replication, thereby blocking virus proliferation.[16,17] The final stage of viral replication is the translation of viral RNA into viral proteins and the self-assembly of viral particles to form a new viron. 1-deoxynojirimycin(DNJ) is an alpha-glucosidase inhibitor against the hepatitis B virus (HBV) that interferes with viral protein glycosylation.[18]

7.6 NANOPARTICLES AS ANTIVIRAL AGENTS AND AS A DRUG DELIVERY SYSTEM

Over the last decade, nanoparticles have played various roles as drug carriers, detection agents, and inhibitory agents against bacteria and viruses. Nanoparticles can act as antiviral agents as well as antiviral drug delivery systems. Nanoparticles

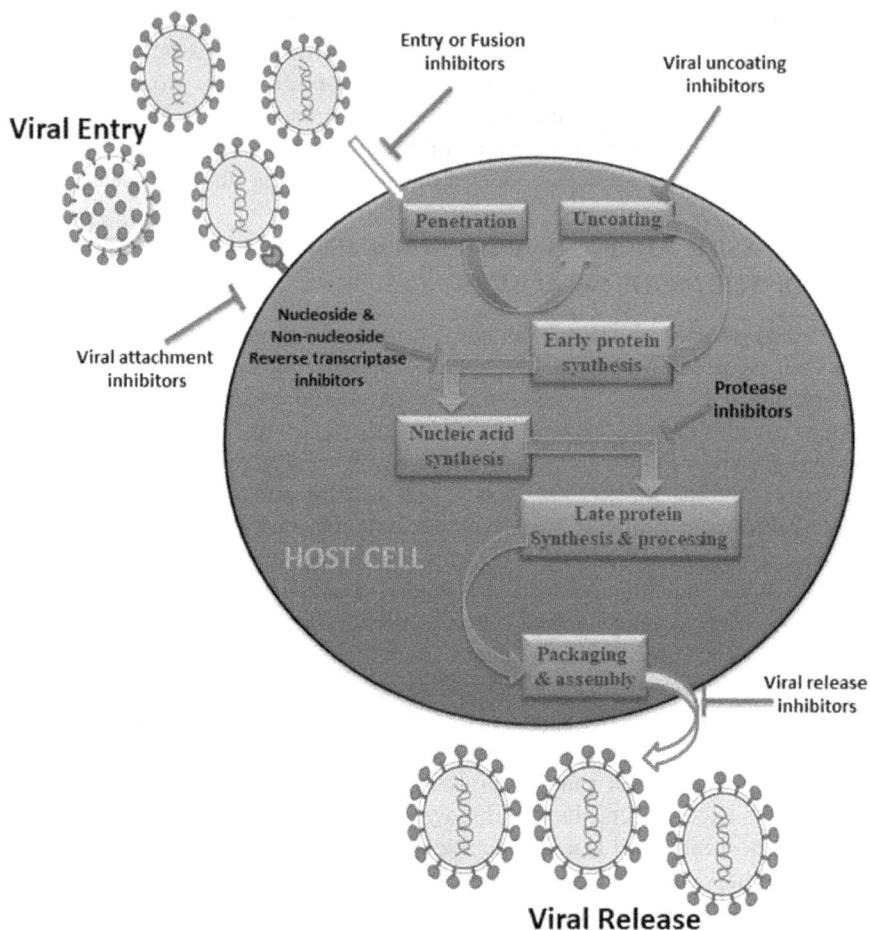

FIGURE 7.2 Intervention strategies to inhibit the different stages of the viral replication cycle.

including gold NPs (AuNPs), silver nanoparticles (AgNPs), carbon dots (CDots), quantum dots (QDs), graphene oxide (GO), silicon materials, polymeric NPs, and dendrimers possess remarkable antibacterial and antiviral activities. The possible antiviral mechanisms include direct or indirect inactivation of a virus, altering capsid protein, preventing virus attachment to host cells, or inhibiting viral replication. Nanoparticles with long flexible linkers mimic heparin sulphate proteoglycans and avoid virus attachment to host cells by competitive inhibition.[19] Nanoparticles adsorbed on the cell surface could alter the membrane potential, blocking virus penetration. Another suggested mechanism is the inactivation of viruses before entry by interaction with DNA or with viral proteins. Inhibition of hemagglutinin and neuraminidase activities may be another possible antiviral mechanism adopted by nanoparticles. Nanoparticle drug formulations are effective in pulmonary drug delivery, which is highly relevant in the COVID-19 pandemic.

Herein, we discuss the various nano-therapies and nano-mediated combination therapy (nanoparticles plus antiviral drugs) for the effective treatment and drug delivery systems for viral infections.

7.6.1 INORGANIC NANOPARTICLES

7.6.1.1 Silver Nanoparticles (AgNPs)

Silver nanoparticles possess unique properties concerning chemical stability, high conductivity, and localized surface plasma resonance, thus making them suitable for biomedical therapeutics. AgNPs have antiviral activity against human parainfluenza, HBV, HIV, HSV, influenza, human oncogenicγ-herpes, and Epstein-Barr and Kaposi's sarcoma-associated herpes viruses.[20-22] AgNPs bind to glycoprotein gp120 on the envelope of the HIV-1 virus and prevent further viral transmission.[23] The discovery of AgNP-coated polyurethane condoms (PUCs) reduced sexually transmitted infections by directly inactivating the HSV-1/2 and HIV-1[24] viruses. Similarly, AgNPs reduced the infection rate of HSV-1/2 and human parainfluenza virus type 3 in a size-dependent manner.[25]

The antiviral activity of AgNPs and chitosan against the H1N1 influenza A virus was more effective in combination than either of them alone.[26] Similarly, the graphene oxide (GO)–AgNP combination was found to be effective against infectious bursal disease virus (IBDV) and feline CoV (FCoV) infections.[27] AgNPs with oseltamivir showed anti-H1N1 activity by interfering with the ROS-mediated signalling pathway by inhibiting neuraminidase and hemagglutinin activity.[28]

7.6.1.2 Gold Nanoparticles (AuNPs)

AuNPs, due to their therapeutic activity, are widely accepted and have excellent optical, electrical, mechanical, and biological properties. Biogenic gold NPs synthesized using green chemistry with seaweed *Sargassum wightii* were reported to have antiviral activity against HSV1, and HSV2 strains.[29] Functionalized AuNPs, including dendronized AuNps and sialic acid, suppress HIV, the influenza virus, and HSV infection.[30] A GNR-5'PPP-ssRNA nanoplex-mediated immune activator or Gold nanorod decreases influenza A (H1N1) viral replication by regulating the expression of IFN-stimulated genes.[31] AuNPs reduces the mRNA expression of interleukin-1β, IL-6, TNF-α, IFN-γ, and inducible nitric oxide synthase.[32] Gold nanoclusters (AuNCs) reported inhibiting the proliferation and protein expression of porcine reproductive and respiratory syndrome virus (PRRSV) in host cells.[33] Halder et al. (2018) showed that highly monodispersed gold nanoparticles stabilized by gallic acid could selectively inhibit HSV by preventing viral cell attachment and penetration with a better safety profile than Acyclovir.[34]

AuNP has also demonstrated the ability to enter various cell types like macrophages, lymphocytes, and brain micro endothelial cells and hence can act as a suitable antiviral delivery system. AuNP conjugated with a lower dose of modified raltegravir inhibited HIV replication after penetrating inside infected PBMCs depleted from CD8+.[35] Paul et al. (2014) proved that the siRNA and AuNP complex had enhanced stability and could reduce the dengue virus replication and release the infectious virion.[36] Peptide-conjugated AuNps exhibit irreversible HIV inactivation by multivalent conjugation with envelope spike proteins.[37] These are less prone to resistance development than synthetic drugs like zanamivir and oseltamivir. Gold and silver nanoparticles could effectively deliver the antiviral peptide FluPep[38] and can be considered an effective strategy for providing therapeutic peptides.

7.6.1.3 Zinc Oxide

Metal oxide particles like ZnO and MgO are considered biocompatible nanoparticles with degradable by-products and are utilized as trace elements in biotherapeutics.[39] *In vivo* studies with zinc oxide tetrapod nanoparticles (ZOTEN) showed clinical improvement in vaginal HSV-2 infection. It presents the virus to mucosal antigen-presenting cells (APCs) and boosts antibody and T cell-mediated immune response to suppress viral activity.[40] ZnO nanoparticles were found to be effective against influenza A (H1N1) virus infection.[41] They also proved that the PEGylated ZnO nanoparticles showed a better inhibition rate than unPEGylated. In vitro studies have reported that ZnO nanoparticles could inhibit SARS-CoV replication.[42]

7.6.2 CARBON-BASED NANOPARTICLES

7.6.2.1 Quantum Dots (QDs)

Quantum dots (QDs) are nanotubes or nanocrystals with 2–10nm diameters made of semiconductor materials. They are a promising drug carrier system due to their stable nature, bioavailability, increased circulation time, active targeting, and localized therapy. Studies have demonstrated that when conjugated with QDs, saquinavir could cross the blood-brain barrier and was effective against HIV.[43] GSH-capped cadmium telluride QDs inhibited viral entry into the cells by altering the surface protein of the pseudorabies virus (PRV).[44] Fluorescent quantum dots allow easy and rapid viral detection and aid in diagnostic purposes. The development of fluorescent quantum dot-conjugated RNA aptamers is suitable for detecting even 0.1 pg.ml−1 concentration of SARS-CoV nucleocapsid protein.[45]

Biomolecule-stabilized carbon quantum dots (CQDs) are more effective and stable. 3-ethoxypropylamine (EPA) and 2,2'-(ethylenedioxy) bis(ethylamine) (EDA) surface-functionalized CQDs were found to be effective against human norovirus virus-like-particles (VLPs) by inhibiting its binding to histo-blood group antigen (HBGA) receptors on human cells.[46] Curcumin stabilized cationic carbon dots are reported to be effective against enterovirus 71 (EV71) and the porcine epidemic diarrhoea virus (PEDV) by changing the viral surface proteins and generating reactive oxygen species (ROS), thereby inducing the production of IFN-stimulated proinflammatory cytokines.[47,48] Further, hydrothermal carbonization of ethylenediamine/citric acid-derived carbon quantum dots (CQDs) interacted well with the viral entry receptors when postmodified with boronic acid ligands. They are considered suitable for the treatment of human coronavirus HCoV-229E infections.[49]

7.6.2.2 Fullerenes

Fullerenes are carbon-based nanostructures and exhibit low cytotoxicity but are less soluble in water. A diamino diacid diphenyl fulleroid is mainly associated with HIV antiviral drug delivery. Buckminsterfullerene (C60), or buckyball, is the most common form and is active against HIV-1, HIV-2, and HCV.[50,51] Significant antiviral activity by fullerene derivatives against influenza A(H1N1), respiratory syncytial virus, Zika virus, and dengue virus was detected.[52]

7.6.2.3 Graphene Oxide

Graphene oxide possesses sharp edges, and its negative charge allows electrostatic interaction, thereby causing increased binding and increased efficacy against viral particles. It also causes the photodegradation of viruses. When irradiated under visible light, graphene tungsten oxide composite film inactivates viruses due to the photodegradation of viral capsid protein.[53] Graphene oxide activity can be enhanced by silver and was found to be effective against other coronavirus variations, including the infectious bursal disease virus and feline coronavirus. Hypericin-loaded graphene oxide complex inhibited viral replication and is advantageous owing to its low cytotoxicity and high loading capacity.[54] The broad-spectrum antiviral compound curcumin limits its application due to low solubility and biocompatibility issues. Curcumin-loaded graphene oxide nanoparticles functionalized with sulfonate group mimic cell surface and prevent viral attachment.[55] GO alone or nanocomposites showed antiviral activity against endemic gastrointestinal avian influenza A virus H9N2, hand-foot-and-mouth disease, EV71, and HSV1.[56,57] GO when conjugated with QDs showed potential inhibition against HIV replication.[58]

7.6.3 Organic Nanoparticles

7.6.3.1 Polymeric Nanoparticles

Polymers are effective antiviral agents or cofactors due to their flexible molecular design. Polymer drug conjugates increase the drug solubility, allowing prolonged retention time, and enhancing the uptake of drugs to cells. Polymeric nanoparticles are synthesized using natural or synthetic polymers and are biocompatible with reduced cytotoxicity. Polymer like poly-D, L-lactic acid, polyglycolic acid, poly-e-caprolactone, and polymethyl methacrylate is approved for human purpose by the United States Food and Drug Administration. A PEG-coated microsphere with acyclovir could be suitable for ocular viral infection treatment. Cidofovir, active against smallpox virus and HCMV was successfully encapsulated in poly(isobutyl cyanoacrylate) nanocapsules.[59] Acyclovir (ACV)-Eudragit (EUD) nanoparticles (NPs) oral bioavailability was found to be higher in human volunteers when compared to commercial ACV tablets.[60] It was observed that Polyhexylcyanoacrylate nanoparticles loaded with Zalcitabine or Saquinavir resulted in a dose-dependent reduction of HIV-1 antigen production.[61] Novel liver-targeted cyclosporine A-encapsulated PLGA nanoparticles were shown to reduce the immunosuppressive effect and toxicity profile of host factor cyclophilin A and inhibit HCV replication.[62] Amphiphilic copolymers encompassing methoxy-poly(ethylene glycol)-block poly(phenylalanine) polymersomes encapsulating mir-323a in the core and favipiravir in the exterior served as an efficient treatment for influenza A viral infections.[63] The chitosan-based biopolymeric nanoparticle is the most focused because of multi-delivery mechanisms suitable for pulmonary drug delivery.[64] Bioavanta-Bosti has developed Novochizol™ to generate intra-pulmonary drug delivery formulations apt for treating COVID-19 patients.

7.6.3.2   Dendrimers

Dendrimers are polymeric nanostructures with a central core and highly branched emanates. They are small with less than 100nm diameter and bind to different ligands, thus making them an attractive drug delivery system. Due to their limited cavity size, dendrimers can encapsulate hydrophobic drugs and can be used to deliver DNA and siRNA, and be effectively used in antiviral therapeutics. VivaGel is the widely known dendrimer used for antiviral therapy against HIV and HSV.[65] It is the first topical nanomicrobicide formed from the divalent l-lysine benzhydylamine amide and contains 32 sodium 1-carboxymethoxynaphthalene-3,6-di-sulphonate as a terminal anionic group which allows the prolonged duration of antiviral activity. A peptide-derived dendrimer SB105 A10 inhibits human cytomegalovirus (HCMV) replication by attaching to the host cell through interaction with heparan sulphate proteoglycans, thereby blocking virion attachment to target cells.[66] Similarly, a complementary combination of carbosilane dendrimers, tenofovir, and maraviroc was found to inhibit the sexual transmission of HIV infection effectively.[67] Polyanionic and cationic dendrimers were shown to have efficient antiviral activity against MERS-CoV plaque formation.[68]

7.6.3.3   Lipid Polymers

Lipid polymer-based drug delivery systems are efficient vehicles for mRNA therapeutics. Lipid nanoparticles like N1, N3, N5-tris(2-aminoethyl) benzene-1,3,5 tricarboxamides along with PLGAs are efficient in antiviral mRNA delivery.[69] Liposomes are a subset of lipid polymers that prefer neutral or negative charge for entrapment efficacy and phagocytosis prevention. When negatively charged liposomes loaded with zidovudine accumulate in essential organs like the spleen and become more effective antiviral therapy.[70] Liposomes are used as a controlled release drug delivery system for Interferons. They improve the serum stability of IFN-α and IFN-γ and have higher immunomodulatory and antiviral efficiency with reduced toxicity.[71] Polyunsaturated liposomes reduce the infectivity of HIV and HCV by suppressing membrane cholesterol levels.[72] Epaxal® and Inflexal® are virosomes (150nm spherical liposomal vesicles) approved as intramuscular vaccine with reduced toxicity and superior immune responses against HAV and influenza, respectively.[73, 74]

7.6.3.4   Micelles and Microemulsions

Micelles and microemulsions are surfactant-based nanoparticles used to formulate a thermodynamically stable drug delivery system. Hydrophobic drugs can be incorporated into their interiors, amphiphilic drugs into their interfacial regions, and hydrophilic drugs encapsulated in reverse micelles or water-in-oil type micro-emulsions. Microemulsions formulated from Tween80, Span 20, isopropyl myristate, oil, and ethanol/water were reported to exhibit activity against HSV-2.[75] Optimized microemulsions effectively suppressed skin lesions caused by HSV in vivo mice models. The antiviral activity of olive leaf extract was enhanced by encapsulating it with O/W microemulsions, and it is hypothesized to inhibit viral attachment to host cell receptors.[76]

7.6.3.5 Nanoemulsions

Nanoemulsions are relatively small droplet emulsions (< 200 nm) with great poten-tial for encapsulation and delivery of antivirals. Natural antivirals like coumestrol, genistein, and curcumin encapsulated in nanoemulsions work effectively against HSV and HPV infections.[77,78] The antiviral drug acyclovir encapsulated in W/O/W nanoemulsions enhances its ability to penetrate the skin.[79] Anti-HIV drugs are less permeable to the blood-brain barrier; hence drug saquinavir mesylate was emulsi-fied in O/W emulsion and delivered via nasal mucosa.[80] Similarly, indinavir in O/W nanoemulsion could cross the blood-brain barrier when administered intravenously.[81] Nanoemulsions have also been effective in intravenous monoclonal antibody delivery in humanized mice.[82] The Self-Nano Emulsifying Drug delivery system (SNEEDS) is a lipid-based monotropic system used for several antiviral drugs like Lauroglycol 90, Capryol 90, or Capmul MCM to improve its penetrative capabilities and bioavail-ability. When the anti-HIV drug Nevirapine was synthesized as SNEEDS, it released 98.9% in the aqueous portion of the GIT, which is a remarkable improvement in the released dosage.[83]

7.7   COMBINATIONAL ANTIVIRAL THERAPY

Combinational antiviral therapy is a widely accepted strategy to improve drug effi-cacy and reduce the risk of drug resistance emerging among mutation-prone viruses. In the late 1990s, the use of antiviral cocktail therapy was highly effective in sup-pressing viral load at different stages of HIV-infected patients.[84,85] Recently combi-national therapies, including antibodies, cytokines, and small molecules, have been recommended to treat COVID-19 patients.[86, 87] Combining antiviral drugs and nano-carriers provided the opportunity to deliver multiple drugs in a safer and controlled manner, thereby reducing drug overdosing and its further complexity.[88] Several com-binational antiviral PLGA nanoparticles are used to treat HIV-1 infections.[89–91]

7.8   NANOPARTICLES TO TACKLE COVID-19

Two nanoparticle-based antivirals, lactoferrin liposomes, and remdesivir, targeting viral replication and reducing inflammation, are undergoing anti-COVID-19 clini-cal trials. Several drugs, including favipiravir, remdesivir, lopinavir/ritonavir, and interferon α (IFN-α), have been used to treat COVID-19. Biopolymeric nanoparticles can be used to deliver these drugs with low toxicity, enhanced solubility, and bio-availability. Chitosan nanoparticles allow pulmonary drug delivery for COVID-19 treatment.[92] Novochizol™ developed by Bioavanta-Bosti to generate intra-pulmonary drug delivery formulations is apt for treating COVID-19 patients. A set of lipid nanoparticle-based mRNA vaccines is under clinical trials for COVID-19. The FDA already approves MRNA-1273 by ModernaTX, Inc, and BNT162b2 by BioNTech SE and Pfizer. A simple, easy-to-handle RNA extraction method was developed using magnetic nanoparticles to detect SARS-Cov-2.[93] Magnetic NPs biosensors are considered promising alternatives for COVID-19 diagnosis. Multi-functional polymeric nanocarriers approved for clinical application could be updated immediately for practical use in the current COVID-19 pandemic.

7.9 NANOPARTICLE-CONJUGATED ANTIVIRALS: ADVANTAGES AND DISADVANTAGES

Successful delivery of antiviral analogs utilizing the prodrug chemistry needs to overcome delivery barriers and challenges, such as poor pharmacokinetics of drugs, low cellular uptake, and unwanted off-target effect. To this effect, due to the structural and morphological resemblance to natural virions, nanocarriers can act as a robust platform that could directly release the drug at the site targeted by viruses. The additional advantages of nanocarriers are constant drug release activity and optimization for multidrug delivery. Enhancing the functional targets of nanocarriers may further broaden the design of antivirals and profoundly eradicate the existing shortcomings of the current antiviral therapeutic regimen. However, several challenges like functional specificity, toxicity, stability, degradation of functional nanoparticles, cost, and production scalability need to be faced while developing nanoparticle-based drugs. Several studies have also reported the inhibitory effects of nanoparticles on drug-resistant viral strains.

7.10 ADVANCEMENTS IN NANOMEDICINE

Nanoscience will become more advanced in the delivery of drug therapy as pharmaceutical research and innovation continue. Better drug delivery systems like nanotraps, nanorobots, etc pave the way to better diagnosis and therapeutics against different viral infections. Nanomedicines including Fluquit (a polymer-based nanotherapeutic with siRNA targeting H5N1, H1N1 Influenza, H7N9), Cervisil (nano-based siRNA formulation for HPV16 and HPV18), DermaVir vaccine for anti-HIV treatment, Doravirine (a next-generation NNRTI for HIV), and Lipid nanoparticles (ARB-001467 TKM-HBV) containing RNAi therapeutics targeting HBV genome are some of the nano drugs currently undergoing various phases of clinical trials. Low-cost cell-friendly multivalent nanogels developed recently also exhibited broad-spectrum antiviral activity by blocking viral entry.[94] Developing hybrid nanoparticles by combining the beneficial attributes of various nanoparticles could create more effective antiviral delivery systems. Bioinspired and biomimetic approaches inspired by natural antimicrobial surfaces are gaining more attention nowadays. More studies are required to explore the diverse and versatile nano molecules to place nanomedicine at the forefront of therapeutics to manage viral infections efficiently.

Nanotechnology needs to be exploited more in the field of diagnostics and imaging. A microelectromechanical system (MEMS) can mimic the secretion of insulin, hormones, and other closed systems. The quantum dots in imaging and diagnosis will continue to develop for advancement in the future. Nanoparticles should be implemented as contrast agents in computed tomography, positron emission tomography (PET), and MRI. In clinical practice, nano-based antiviral therapy and diagnostics should be encouraged to make treatment more cost-effective, low cytotoxic, and high-quality formulations for precise treatment.

7.11   CONCLUSION

Viral infections pose a serious global public health and economic threat, as demonstrated by the recent COVID-19 pandemic. Even though many antivirals are already available, numerous challenges limit their efficacy. With the recent advancement in nanotechnology, we can overcome the problems in antiviral therapy development by identifying and developing appropriate nano-based drugs in addition to conventional strategies. To some extent, the emergence of drug resistance, a major upcoming problem in drug development, can be addressed using nanoparticles. Nanotechnology also plays a significant role in viral disease diagnosis, therapeutics, and biomedical applications. Even though the progress of nanotechnology in the development of antiviral therapy is in its infancy, there are great expectations for the development of better therapeutic strategies to combat future pandemics.

REFERENCES

1. World Health Organisation. (2020) Statement on the second meeting of the international health regulations (2005), emergency committee regarding the outbreak of novel coronavirus (2019-nCoV). https://www.who.int/news-room/detail/30-01-2020-statement-on-the-second-meeting-of-the-international-healthregulations-(2005)-emergency-committee-regarding-the-outbreak-of-novel-coronavirus-(2019-ncov).
2. Grubaugh, N.D., Ladner, J.T., Lemey, P., Pybus, O.G., Rambaut, A., Holmes, E.C., Andersen, K.G. (2019) Tracking virus outbreaks in the twenty-first century. *Nat. Microbiol.* 4(1), 10–19. https://doi.org/10.1038/s41564-018-0296-2.
3. World Health Organisation (WHO). (2018) R&D Blueprint, about the R&D. *Blueprint.* https://www.who.int/blueprint/about/en/.
4. Fitzgerald, J.G. (1911) Ehrlich-Hata remedy for Syphilis. *Can. Med. Assoc. J.* 1(1), 38–46.
5. Domagk, G. (1950) Sulfonamides in the past, present and future. *Minerva. Med.* 35(35), 41–47.
6. Porrit, A.E. (1951) The discovery development of penicillin. *Med. Press* 19, 460–462.
7. Adamson, C.S., Chibale, K., Goss, R.J.M., Jaspars, M., Newman, D.J., Dorrington, R.A. (2021) Antiviral drug discovery: Preparing for the next pandemic. *Chem. Soc. Rev.* 50(6), 3647–3655.
8. Ison, M.G. (2011) Antivirals and resistance: Influenza virus. *Curr. Opin. Virol.* 1(6), 563–573.
9. Moore, J.P., Stevenson, M. (2000) New targets for inhibitors of HIV-1 replication. *Nat. Rev. Mol. Cell Biol.* 1(1), 40–49.

10. Blaas, D. (2016) Viral entry pathways: The example of common cold viruses. *Wien. Med. Wochenschr.* 166(7–8), 211–226.

11. Hubsher, G., Haider, M., Okun, M.S. (2012) Amantadine: The journey from fighting flu to treating Parkinson's disease. *Neurology* 78(14), 1096–1099.

12. Saito, R., Li, D., Sato, M., Suzuki, H. (2006) Amantadine. *Virus Rep.* 3(1), 40–47.

13. Fleming, D.M. (2001) Managing influenza: Amantadine, rimantadine and beyond. *Int. J. Clin. Pract.* 55(3), 189–195.

14. Hayden, F.G. (1996) Amantadine and rimantadine—Clinical aspects. In: *Antiviral Drug Resistance*; Richman, D.D., Ed.; Wiley,New York pp. 59–77.

15. Hay, A.J. (1996) Amantadine and rimantadine-mechanisms. In: *Antiviral Drug Resistance*; Richman, D.D., Ed.; Wiley, New York pp. 43–58.

16. Gao, Y., Yan, L., Huang, Y., Liu, F., Zhao, Y., Cao, L., et al. (2020) Structure of the RNA-dependent RNA polymerase from COVID-19 virus. *Science* 368(6492), 779–782.

17. Yin, W., Mao, C., Luan, X., Shen, D.D., Shen, Q., Su, H., et al. (2020) Structural basis for inhibition of the RNA-dependent RNA polymerase from SARS-CoV-2 by remdesivir. *Science* 368(6498), 1499–1504.

18. Jacob, J.R., Mansfeld, K., You, J.E., Tennant, B.C., Kim, Y.H. (2007) Natural iminosugar derivatives of 1-deoxynojirimycin inhibit glycosylation of hepatitis viral envelope proteins. *J. Microbiol.* 45(5), 431–440.

19. Cagno, V., Andreozzi, P., D'Alicarnasso, M., Silva, P.J., Mueller, M., Galloux, M., et al. (2018) Broad-spectrum non-toxic antiviral nanoparticles with a virucidal inhibition mechanism. *Nat. Mater.* 17(2), 195–203.

20. Huy, T.Q., Hien Thanh, N.T., Thuy, N.T., Van Chung, P., Hung, P.N., Le, A.T., et al. (2017) Cytotoxicity and antiviral activity of electrochemical—Synthesized silver nanoparticles against poliovirus. *J. Virol. Methods* 241, 52–57.

21. Xiang, D., Zheng, C., Zheng, Y., Li, X., Yin, J., O'Conner, M., et al. (2013) Inhibition of A/Human/Hubei/3/2005 (H3N2) influenza virus infection by silver nanoparticles in vitro and in vivo. *Int. J. Nanomed.* 8, 4103.

22. Wan, C., Tai, J., Zhang, J., Guo, Y., Zhu, Q., Ling, D., et al. (2019) Silver nanoparticles selectively induce human oncogenicγ-herpesvirus-related cancer cell death through reactivating viral lytic replication. *Cell Death Dis.* 10(6), 1–16.

23. Lara, H.H., Ayala-Nuñez, N.V., Ixtepan-Turrent, L., Rodriguez-Padilla, C. (2010) Mode of antiviral action of silver nanoparticles against HIV-1. *J. Nanobiotechnol.* 8, 1–10.

24. Mohammed Fayaz, M.A., Ao, Z., Girilal, M., Chen, L., Xiao, X., Kalaichelvan, P.T., et al. (2012) Inactivation of microbial infectiousness by silver nanoparticles-coated condom: A new approach to inhibit HIV– and HSV-transmitted infection. *Int. J. Nanomed.* 7, 5007–5018.

25. Gaikwad, S., Ingle, A., Gade, A., Rai, M., Falanga, A., Incoronato, N., et al. (2013) Antiviral activity of my synthesized silver nanoparticles against herpes simplex virus and human parainfluenza virus type 3. *Int. J. Nanomed.* 8, 4303–4314.

26. Lv, X., Wang, P., Bai, R., Cong, Y., Suo, S., Ren, X., et al. (2014) Inhibitory effect of silver nanomaterials on transmissible virus-induced host cell infections. *Biomaterials* 35(13), 4195–4203.

27. Chen, Y.N., Hsueh, Y.H., Hsieh, C.T., Tzou, D.Y., Chang, P.L. (2016) Antiviral activity of graphene–silvernanocomposites against non-enveloped and enveloped viruses. *Int. J. Environ. Res. Public Health* 13(4), 430.

28. Li, Y., Lin, Z., Zhao, M., Xu, T., Wang, C., Hua, L., et al. (2016) Silver nanoparticle based codelivery of oseltamivir to inhibit the activity of the H1N1 influenza virus through ROS-mediated signaling pathways. *ACS Appl. Mater. Interfaces* 8(37), 24385–24393.

29. Singaravelu, G., Arockiamary, J.S., Kumar, V.G., Govindaraju, K. (2007) A novel extracellular synthesis of monodisperse gold nanoparticles using marine alga, Sargassum wightii Greville. *Colloids Surf.* 57(1), 97–101.

30. Papp, I., Sieben, C., Ludwig, K., Roskamp, M., Böttcher, C., Schlecht, S., et al. (2010) Inhibition of influenza virus infection by multivalent sialic-acid- functionalized gold nanoparticles. *Small* 6(24), 2900–2906.

31. Chakravarthy, K.V., Bonoiu, A.C., Davis, W.G., Ranjan, P., Ding, H., Hu, R., et al. (2010) Gold nanorod delivery of an ssRNA immune activator inhibits pandemic H1N1 influenza viral replication. *Proc. Natl. Acad. Sci. U. S. A.* 107(22), 10172–10177.

32. Dkhil, M.A., Bauomy, A.A., Diab, M.S., Al-Quraishy, S. (2015) Antioxidant and hepatoprotective role of gold nanoparticles against murine hepatic schistosomiasis. *Int. J. Nanomed.* 10, 7467.

33. Bai, Y., Zhou, Y., Liu, H., Fang, L., Liang, J., Xiao, S. (2018) Glutathione-stabilized fluorescent gold nanoclusters vary in their influences on the proliferation of pseudorabies virus and porcine reproductive and respiratory syndrome virus. *ACS Appl. Nano Mater.* 1(2), 969–976.

34. Halder, A., Das, S., Ojha, D., Chattopadhyay, D., Mukherjee, A. (2018) Highly monodispersed gold nanoparticles synthesis and inhibition of herpes simplex virus infections. *Mater. Sci. Eng. C Mater. Biol. Appl.* 89, 413–421.

35. Bayo, J.M.P.D., Martinez, E. (2015) Medicinal chemistry. *Future Med. Chem.* 7, 450–461.

36. Paul, A.M., Shi, Y., Acharya, D., Douglas, J.R., Cooley, A., Anderson, J.F., et al. (2014) Delivery of antiviral small interfering RNA with gold nanoparticles inhibits dengue virus infection in vitro. *J. Gen. Virol.* 95(8), 1712–1722.

37. Bastian, A.R., Nangarlia, A., Bailey, L.D., Holmes, A., Sundaram, R.V.K., Ang, C., et al. (2015) Mechanism of multivalent nanoparticle encounter with HIV-1 for potency enhancement of peptide triazole virus inactivation. *J. Biol. Chem.* 290(1), 529–543.

38. Alghrair, Z.K., Fernig, D.G., Bahram, E. (2019) Enhanced inhibition of influenza virus infection by peptide-noble-metal nanoparticle conjugates. *Beilstein J. Nanotechnol.* 10, 1038–1047.

39. Zhang, R., Liu, X., Xiong, Z., Huang, Q., Yang, X., Yan, H., et al. (2018) Novel micro/nanostructured TiO_2/ZnO coating with antibacterial capacity and cytocompatibility. *Ceram. Int.* 44(8), 9711–9719.

40. Antoine, T.E., Hadigal, S.R., Yakoub, A.M., Mishra, Y.K., Bhattacharya, P., Haddad, C., et al. (2016) Intravaginal zinc oxide tetrapod nanoparticles as novel immunoprotective agents against genital herpes. *J. Immunol.* 196(11), 4566–4575.

41. Ghaffari, H., Tavakoli, A., Moradi, A., Tabarraei, A., Bokharaei-Salim, F., Zahmatkeshan, M. et al. (2019) Inhibition of H1N1 influenza virus infection by zinc oxide nanoparticles: Another emerging application of nanomedicine. *J. Biomed. Sci.* 26(1), 70.

42. Te Velthuis, A.J.W., van den Worm, S.H.E., Sims, A.C., Baric, R.S., Snijder, E.J., van Hemert, M.J. (2010) Zn(2+) inhibits coronavirus and Arterivirus RNA polymerase activity in vitro and zinc ionophores block the replication of these viruses in cell culture. *PLOS Pathog.* 6(11), e1001176.

43. Yong, K., Wang, Y., Roy, I., Rui, H., Swihart, M.T., Law, W., et al. (2012) Preparation of quantum dot/drug nanoparticle formulations for traceable targeted delivery and therapy. *Theranostics* 2(7), 681.

44. Du, T., Cai, K., Han, H., Fang, L., Liang, J., Xiao, S. (2015) Probing the interactions of CdTe quantum dots with pseudorabies virus. *Sci. Rep.* 5, 1–10.

45. Roh, C., Jo, S.K. (2011) Quantitative and sensitive detection of SARS coronavirus nucleocapsid protein using quantum dots-conjugated RNA aptamer on chip. *J. Chem. Technol. Biotechnol.* 86(12), 1475–1479.

46. Dong, X., Moyer, M.M., Yang, F., Sun, Y.P., Yang, L. (2017) Carbon dots' antiviral functions against noroviruses. *Sci. Rep.* 7(1), 1–10.

47. Du, T., Liang, J., Dong, N., Lu, J., Fu, Y., Fang, L., et al. (2018) Glutathione-capped Ag2S nanoclusters inhibit coronavirus proliferation through blockage of viral RNA synthesis and budding. *ACS Appl. Mater. Interfaces* 10(5), 4369–4378.

48. Lin, C., Chang, L., Chu, H., Lin, H., Chang, P., Wang, R.Y.L., et al. (2019) High amplification of the antiviral activity of curcumin through transformation into carbon quantum dots. *Small* 15(41), 1902641.

49. Łoczechin, A., Séron, K., Barras, A., Giovanelli, E., Belouzard, S., Chen, Y., et al. (2019) Functional carbon quantum dots as medical countermeasures to human coronavirus. *ACS Appl. Mater. Interfaces* 11(46), 42964–42974.

50. Bosi, S., Da Ros, T., Spalluto, G., Balzarini, J., Prato, M. (2003) Synthesis andanti-HIV properties of new water-soluble bis-functionalized[60]fullerene derivatives. *Bioorg. Med. Chem. Lett.* 13(24), 4437–4440.

51. Mashino, T., Shimotohno, K., Ikegami, N., Nishikawa, D., Okuda, K., Takahashi, K., et al. (2005) Human immunodeficiency virus-reverse transcriptase inhibition and hepatitis C virus RNA-dependent RNA polymerase inhibition activities of fullerene derivatives. *Bioorg. Med. Chem. Lett.* 15(4), 1107–1109.

52. Innocenzi, P., Stagi, L. (2020) Carbon-based antiviral nanomaterials: Graphene, C-dots, and fullerenes: A perspective. *Chem. Sci.* 11(26), 6606–6622.

53. Akhavan, O., Choobtashani, M., Ghaderi, E. (2012) Protein degradation and RNA efflux of viruses photocatalyzed by graphene–tungsten oxide composite under visible light irradiation. *J. Phys. Chem. C* 116(17), 9653–9659.

54. Du, X., Xiao, R., Fu, H., Yuan, Z., Zhang, W., Yin, L., et al. (2019) Hypericin-loaded graphene oxide protects ducks against a novel duck reovirus. *Mater. Sci. Eng. C Mater. Biol. Appl.* 105, 110052.

55. Yang, X.X., Li, C.M., Li, Y.F., Wang, J., Huang, C.Z. (2017) Synergistic antiviral effect of curcumin functionalized graphene oxide against respiratory syncytial virus infection nanoscale 9(41), 16086–16092.

56. Song, Z., Wang, X., Zhu, G., Nian, Q., Zhou, H., Yang, D., et al. (2015) Virus capture and destruction bylabel-free graphene oxide for detection and disinfection applications. *Small* 11(9–10), 1171–1176.

57. Sametband, M., Kalt, I., Gedanken, A., Sarid, R. (2014) Herpes simplex virus type-1 attachment inhibition by functionalized graphene oxide. *ACS Appl. Mater. Interfaces* 6(2), 1228–1235.

58. Iannazzo, D., Pistone, A., Salamò, M., Galvagno, S., Romeo, R., Giofré, S.V., et al. (2017) Graphene quantum dots for cancer targeted drug delivery. *Int. J. Pharm.* 518(1–2), 185–192.

59. Hillaireau, H., Le Doan, T., Besnard, M., Chacun, H., Janin, J., Couvreur, P. (2006) Encapsulation of antiviral nucleotide analogues azidothymidine-triphosphate and cidofovir in poly(iso-butylcyanoacrylate) nanocapsules. *Int. J. Pharm.* 324(1), 37–42.

60. Elshafeey, A.H., Kamel, A.O., Awad, G.A.S. (2010) Ammonium methacrylate units polymer content and their effect on acyclovir colloidal nanoparticles properties and bioavailability in human volunteers. *Colloids Surf. B Biointerfaces* 75(2), 398–404.

61. Bender, A.R., Von Briesen, H., Kreuter, J., Duncan, I.B., Rubsamen-Waigmann, H. (1996) Efficiency of nanoparticles as a carrier system for antiviral agents in human immunodeficiency virus-infected human monocytes/macrophages in vitro. *Antimicrob. Agents Chemother.* 40(6), 1467–1471.

62. Jyothi, K.R., Beloor, J., Jo, A., Nguyen, M.N., Choi, T.G., Kim, J.H., et al. (2015) Liver-targeted cyclosporine A-encapsulated poly (lactic-co-glycolic) acid nanoparticles inhibit hepatitis C virus replication. *Int. J. Nanomedicine* 10, 903–921.

63. Chun, H., Yeom, M., Kim, H.O., Lim, J.W., Na, W., Park, G., et al. (2018) Efficient antiviral co-delivery using polymersomes by controlling the surface density of cell-targeting groups for influenza A virus treatment. *Polym. Chem.* 9(16), 2116–2123.

64. Rothan, H.A., Byrareddy, S.N. (2020) The epidemiology and pathogenesis of coronavirus disease (COVID-19) outbreak. *J. Autoimmun.* 109, Article 102433.

65. Rupp, R., Rosenthal, S.L., Stanberry, L.R. (2007) VivaGel (SPL7013 Gel): A candidate dendrimer–Microbicide for the prevention of HIV and HSV infection. *Int. J. Nanomedicine* 2(4), 561–566.

66. Luganini, A., Giuliani, A., Pirri, G., Pizzuto, L., Landolfo, S., Gribaudo, G. (2010) Peptide-derivatized dendrimers inhibit human cytomegalovirus infection by blocking virus binding to cell surface heparan sulfate. *Antivir. Res.* 85(3), 532–540.

67. Sepúlveda-Crespo, D., Sánchez-Rodríguez, J., Serramía, M.J., Gómez, R., De La Mata, F.J., Jiménez, J.L., et al. (2015) Triple combination of carbosilane dendrimers, tenofovir and maraviroc as potential microbicide to prevent HIV-1 sexual transmission. *Nanomedicine.* 10(6), 899–914.

68. Kandeel, M., Al-Taher, A., Park, B.K., Kwon, H., Al-Nazawi, M. (2020) A pilot study of the antiviral activity ofanionic and cationic polyamidoamine dendrimers against the Middle East respiratory syndrome coronavirus. *J. Med. Virol.* 92(9), 1665–1670.

69. Zhao, W., Zhang, C., Zhang, X., Luo, X., Zeng, C., Li, W., et al. (2018) Lipid polymer hybrid nanomaterials for mRNA delivery. *Cell. Mol. Bioeng.* 11(5), 397–406.

70. Kaur, C.D., Nahar, M., Jain, N.K. (2008) Lymphatic targeting of zidovudine using surface-engineered liposomes. *J. Drug Target.* 16(10), 798–805.

71. Saravolac, E.G., Kournikakis, B., Gorton, L., Wong, J.P. (1996) Effect of liposome-encapsulation on immunomodulating and antiviral activities of interferon-gamma 1. *Antiviral Res.* 29(2–3), 199–207.

72. Pollock, S., Nichita, N.B., Böhmer, A., Radulescu, C., Dwek, R.A., Zitzmann, N. (2010) Polyunsaturated liposomes are antiviral against hepatitis B and C viruses and HIV by decreasing cholesterol levels in infected cells. *Proc. Natl Acad. Sci. U. S. A.* 107(40), 17176–17181.

73. Bovier, P.A. (2008) Epaxal®: A virosomal vaccine to prevent hepatitis A infection. *Exp. Rev. Vaccines* 7(8), 1141–1150.

74. Herzog, C., Hartmann, K., Künzi, V., Kürsteiner, O., Mischler, R., Lazar, H., et al. (2009) Eleven years of Inflexal®V—A virosomal adjuvanted influenza vaccine.*Vaccine* 27(33), 4381–4387.

75. Alkhatib, M.H., Aly, M.M., Rahbeni, R.A., Balamash, K.S. (2016) Antimicrobial activity of biocompatible microemulsions against Aspergillus niger and herpes simplex virus type 2. *Jundishapur J. Microbiol.* 9(9), e37437.

76. Khattab, R.A., Hosny, A.E., Abdelkawy, M.A., Fahmy, R.H., ElMenoufy, N.A. (2016) Anti-HSV type-1 activity of olive leaves extract crude form acting as a microemulsion dosage form. *Afr. J. Microbiol. Res.* 10(22), 820–828.

77. Argenta, D.F., Bidone, J., Misturini, F.D., Koester, L.S., Bassani, V.L., Simoes, C.M.O., et al. (2016) In vitro evaluation of mucosa permeation/retention and antiherpes activity of genistein from cationic nanoemulsions. *J. Nanosci. Nanotechnol.* 16(2), 1282–1290.

78. do Bonfim, C.M., Monteleoni, L.F., Calmon, M.D., Candido, N.M., Provazzi, P.J.S., Lino, V.D., et al. (2020) Antiviral activity of curcumin-nanoemulsion associated with photodynamic therapy in vulvar cell lines transducing different variants of HPV-16. *Artif. Cells Nanomed. Biotechnol.* 48(1), 515–524.

79. Schwarz, J.C., Klang, V., Karall, S., Mahrhauser, D., Resch, G.P., Valenta, C. (2012) Optimisation of multiple W/O/W nanoemulsions for dermal delivery of acyclovir. *Int. J. Pharm.* 435(1), 69–75.

80. Mahajan, H.S., Mahajan, M.S., Nerkar, P.P., Agrawal, A. (2014) Nanoemulsion-based intranasal drug delivery system of saquinavir mesylate for brain targeting. *Drug Deliv.* 21(2), 148–154.

81. Prabhakar, K., Afzal, S.M., Surender, G., Kishan, V. (2013) Tween 80 containing lipid nanoemulsions for delivery of indinavir to brain. *Acta Pharm. Sin. B* 3(5), 345–353.

82. Pardi, N., Secreto, A.J., Shan, X.C., Debonera, F., Glover, J., Yi, Y.J., et al. (2017) Administration of nucleoside-modified mRNA encoding broadly neutralizing antibody protects humanized mice from HIV-1 challenge. *Nat. Commun.* 8, 14630.

83. Selvam, R., Kulkarni, P. (2014) Design and evaluation of self nanoemulsifying systems for poorly water soluble HIV drug. *J. Pharma.Sci.Tech.* 4, 23–28.

84. Perelson, A.S., Essunger, P., Cao, Y., Vesanen, M., Hurley, A., Saksela, K., et al. (1997) Decay characteristics of HIV-1-infected compartments during combination therapy. *Nature* 387(6629), 188–191.

85. Zhang, L., Ramratnam, B., Tenner-Racz, K., He, Y., Vesanen, M., Lewin, S., et al. (1999) Quantifying residual HIV-1 replication in patients receiving combination antiretroviral therapy. *N. Engl. J. Med.* 340(21), 1605–1613.

86. Wang, W., Xu, Y., Gao, R., Lu, R., Han, K., Wu, G., et al. (2020) Detection of SARS-CoV-2 in diferent types of clinical specimens. *JAMA* 323(18), 1843–1844.

87. Hung, I.F., Lung, K.C., Tso, E.Y., Liu, R., Chung, T.W., Chu, M.Y., et al. (2020) Triple combination of interferon beta-1b, lopinavir-ritonavir, and ribavirin in the treatment of patients admitted to hospital with COVID-19: An open-label, randomised, phase 2 trial. *Lancet* 395(10238), 1695–1704.

88. Freeling, J.P., Koehn, J., Shu, C., Sun, J., Ho, R.J. (2015) Anti-HIV drug combination nanoparticles enhance plasma drug exposure duration as well as triple-drug combination levels in cells within lymph nodes and blood in primates. *AIDS Res. Hum. Retrovir.* 31(1), 107–114.

89. Shibata, A., McMullen, E., Pham, A., Belshan, M., Sanford, B., Zhou, Y., et al. (2013) Polymeric nanoparticles containing combination antiretroviral drugs for HIV type 1 treatment. *AIDS Res. Hum. Retrovir.* 29(5), 746–754.

90. Kumar, P., Lakshmi, Y.S., Kondapi, A.K. (2017) Triple drug combination of zidovudine, efavirenz and lamivudine loaded lactoferrin nanoparticles: An effective nano first-line regimen for HIV therapy. *Pharm. Res.* 34(2), 257–268.

91. Mandal, S., Kang, G., Prathipati, P.K., Fan, W., Li, Q., Destache, C.J. (2018) Long-acting parenteral combination antiretroviral loaded Nano drug delivery system to treat chronic HIV-1 infection: A human ized mouse model study. *Antiviral Res.* 156, 85–91.

92. Chowdhury, N.K., Deepika, C.R., Sonawane, G.A., Mavinamar, S., Lyu, X., Pandey, R.P., et al. (2021) Nanoparticles as an effective drug delivery system in Covid-19. *Biomed. Pharmacother.* 2021, 112162.

93. Zhao, Z., Cui, H., Song, W., Ru, X., Zhou, W., Yu, X.A. (2020) Simple magnetic nanoparticles-based viral RNA extraction method for efficient detection of SARS-CoV-2. *bioRxiv*, 518055. https://doi.org/10.1101/2020.02.22.961268.

94. Dey, P., Bergmann, T., Cuellar-Camacho, J.L., Ehrmann, S., Chowdhury, M.S., Zhang, M., et al. (2018) Multivalent flexible nanogels exhibit broad-spectrum antiviral activity by blocking virus entry. *ACS Nano* 12(7), 6429–6442.

8 Nanotechnology in Antiviral Treatment against Coronavirus

Sasidharan Venkataramanan,
Gad Elsayed Mohamed Salem,
Neetu Talreja, Divya Chauhan,
Mangalaraja Ramalinga Viswanathan,
and Mohammad Ashfaq

CONTENTS

8.1 INTRODUCTION

Presently, several deadly viruses are highlighted that cause death in humans within a short duration of time. These viruses are contagious and deadly enough to destroy a part of the population by attacking their cell, tissue, and subsequently organ. There are two categories of viruses: double-stranded DNA (ds-DNA), poxviruses, herpes viruses, adenoviruses, and single-stranded DNA (ss-DNA) like parvoviruses. There are also some ds-DNA- and ss-RNA-based virus-like reoviruses and the most recent one, severe acute respiratory syndrome coronavirus 2 (SARS-CoV-2), respectively. The virus enters inside the source body and uses six essential steps: (1) attachment, (2) penetration, (3) uncoating, (4) replication, (5) assembly, and (6) release. Several clinical treatments can apply to drugs to treat antiviral diseases, such as acyclovir, ivermectin, ganciclovir, etc. (Chen and Liang, 2020a; Vodnar et al., 2020; Nickels, 2020; Trefry and Wooley, 2012). However, severe side effects limit their application in treatments against the virus. Moreover, several viruses cannot even be treated by drugs or vaccination. In this context, it is necessary to develop novel drugs for the treatment of the virus.

Novel strategies, including emerging nanomaterials (NMs) as a drug against the treatment of the virus, can effectively treat the virus. Several unique properties of NMs such as large surface area, large functional sites, and shape and size tuning properties with biocompatibility allow them to be effectively used as an antiviral drug. Numerous NMs, including carbon-based nanomaterials (CBMs) (CNTs, CNFs, graphene, and graphene oxides), metal-based NMs (Ag, Au, Cu, Fe, and Zn, etc.) have been synthesized and effectively kill or inhibit bacteria and viruses with minimal cytotoxicity. These NMs are attracting wide interest due to their optical, catalytic, electrical, and antimicrobial properties. Transition metal and metal oxide-based nanoparticles are suitable substitutes for noble metals, such as Ag and Au, as these have wider commercial benefits, including their availability, low cost, and highly conductive properties. Furthermore, the properties of these transition metal-based nanomaterials can be easily tuned by changing the synthesis (Ashfaq et al., 2016, 2014, 2013, 2017b; Bhadauriya et al., 2018; Afreen et al., 2018; Sasidharan et al., 2021; Chauhan et al., 2020; Omar et al., 2019b; Ashfaq et al., 2019; Afreen et al., 2020; Ashfaq et al., 2021; Chauhan et al., 2021; Omar et al., 2022; Talreja et al., 2021a, 2021c; Sultana et al., 2021; Mustafa et al., 2011; Chauhan, 2021). Moreover, functionalization using different functional groups of NMs has also been counted as an efficient antiviral candidate (Nickels, 2020; Peplow, 2021; Merkl et al., 2021; Ibrahim Fouad, 2021; Carvalho and Conte-Junior, 2021). Several studies reported the application of these nanomaterials as antiviral agents. For example, Kumar et al. synthesized iron oxide nanoparticles as an antiviral agent. The authors stated that synthesized nanoparticles worked well against the H1N1 influenza A virus (Kumar et al., 2019). Shionoiri et al. synthesized copper iodide nanoparticles to function against feline calicivirus (Shionoiri et al., 2012). Galdiero et al. synthesized silver nanoparticles as an antiviral agent (Galdiero et al., 2011). Another theoretical investigation by Mehranfar et al. was performed over gold nanoparticles to explore the effectiveness against the most recent virus, Severe Acute Respiratory Syndrome Coronavirus 2 (SARS-CoV-2) (Mehranfar and Izadyar, 2020). These studies prove the applicability of nanomaterial as an effective antibacterial and antiviral agent. This chapter focuses on nanotechnology and its applicability to antiviral activity, especially COVID-19 (Figure 8.1).

8.2   SYNTHESIS OF NANOMATERIALS (NMS)

The NMs are synthesized mainly by coprecipitation, sol-gel, hydrothermal, sonochemical, and microwave-assisted based chemical methods. Herein, we explore the different methods of synthesizing, including physical, chemical, and biological, for nanomaterials to effectively apply as an antiviral agent.

8.2.1   COPRECIPITATION PROCESS

Coprecipitation is the simplest method for the synthesis of NMs. In this method, trivalent and divalent salt mix under temperature in a base to form an insoluble salt. The

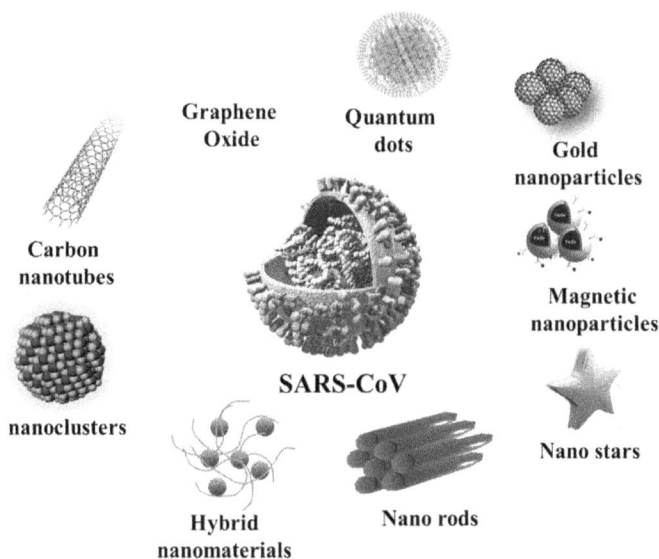

FIGURE 8.1   A graphical representation of various NMs and their antiviral effects.

mechanism behind nanoparticle formation using coprecipitation is that nucleation suddenly appears in solution when reacting salts achieve supersaturation. Subsequently, the growth of this nucleation occurs by diffusion to produce nanoparticles. The shape and size of synthesized nanoparticles usually are controlled by changing the pH, temperature, and salt concentration used. The method generally synthesizes low-quality crystals. However, the crystallinity can be controlled by varying temperatures and reacting, changing the basicity of a solution. Several studies report the synthesis of nanomaterials using the coprecipitation method, including LaGrow et al. synthesizing iron oxide nanoparticles using the coprecipitation method. The authors abruptly change the solution's pH, which subsequently affects the size and crystal quality of iron oxide nanoparticles (LaGrow et al., 2019). Another study by Ashfaq et al. synthesized Fe-Bi povidone-iodine micro composite using the coprecipitation method. The authors utilized the synthesized nanomaterial for the photodegradation of rhodamine and bacteria (Ashfaq et al., 2021). Another study by Ding et al. synthesized $LiFePO_4$/graphene-based composite using the coprecipitation method. The authors improved the crystal quality of the composite by changing the amount of graphene during coprecipitation and utilized the synthesized composite in secondary lithium batteries (Ding et al., 2010). Amighian et al. synthesized manganese ferrite ($MnFe_2O_4$) using the coprecipitation method (Amighian et al., 2006). These studies suggest that coprecipitation is a useful method for controlling crystal quality by varying the temperature and pH of the solution.

8.2.2   Sol-Gel Process

The sol-gel process is extensively used in synthesizing micron-/nano-sized materials and is widely used in different applications due to providing relatively superior enhancement for metallic coating onto the substrate. Usually, the sol-gel process is relatively simple, inexpensive, and has tremendous coating ability on the substrate, thereby it has wider applicability (Hench and West, 1990; Livage, 1997; Parashar et al., 2020; Danks et al., 2016; Alberti and Jágerská, 2021).

8.2.3 Chemical Vapour Deposition (CVD) Process

The CVD process is used to synthesize various nanomaterials like carbon nanofibers (CNFs), carbon nanotubes (CNTs), graphene, etc. Usually, in the CVD process, chemical components react with the vapour phase that is close to the hot substrate. The substrate activates with the temperature or plasma and deposition of powder or coating onto the substrate. The CVD process produces high-quality crystals and has a high yield of nanomaterials (Muñoz and Gómez-Aleixandre, 2013; Schwander and Partes, 2011; Cai et al., 2018; Ani et al., 2018).

8.3 SARS-COVID-19

Coronavirus was first discovered in the 1960s and is considered a most dangerous virus that increases mortality and morbidity rates. Approximately 60% of infectious diseases spread due to zoonoses, and the bat served as a pathogen host that spread infectious diseases to human beings. Numerous coronaviruses (CoV) like the Middle East respiratory syndrome (MERS) CoV, severe acute respiratory syndrome (SARS) CoV 1 (SARS-CoV-1), and SARS-CoV-2 spread through bats. In 2019, a severe pneumonia infection arose in Wuhan, in the Hubei region, China due to an obscure reason. After a few days, this secretive pneumonia infection was recognized as SARS-CoV-2. The threatening infection was named Covid infection 2019 (COVID-19) by the World Health Organization (WHO). The WHO has decreed the outbreak of the novel COVID-19 transported by SARS-CoV-2 that create a global pandemic (Jones et al., 2008; Chauhan, 2021; Rohr et al., 2019; Sharma et al., 2020; Abdelrahman et al., 2020; V'kovski et al., 2021; Park, 2020; Al-Qahtani, 2020; Tang et al., 2020). The COVID-19 pandemic spread from China to other countries rapidly, covering almost all countries worldwide. The transmissions of COVID-19 are not clearly understood. Moreover, several reports suggested that the COVID-19 virus spread through respiratory droplets from direct contact with an infected person or another person (Abdelrahman et al., 2020; Jayaweera et al., 2020; Klompas et al., 2020; Leung, 2021).

The COVID-19 virus depends on the ACE2 receptors' host cell entry as well as replication of the virus. The higher viral loads observed in the respiratory tract indicate the requirement of a repeat test of the suspect patients' upper/lower respiratory tract (initially negative) (Kevadiya et al., 2021; Kragstrup et al., 2021; Proal and VanElzakker, 2021). With the help of nanomaterials, the COVID-19 pandemic might be controlled by using nanomaterial-based masks and drug delivery (Figure 8.2).

8.4 ANTIVIRAL ACTIVITY OF NANOMATERIALS

Viral infections are one of the greatest challenges globally due to their distributing behaviours and their ability to develop through a genetic mutation that causes

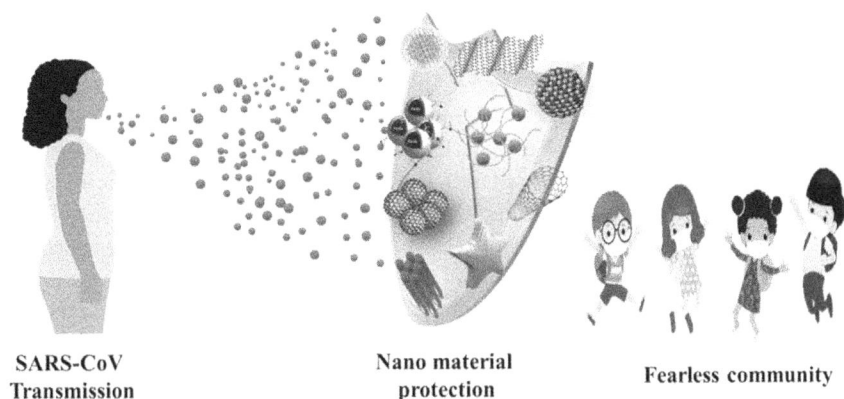

SARS-CoV
Transmission

Nano material
protection

Fearless community

FIGURE 8.2   Schematic illustration of the COVID-19 shield with the help of nanomaterials.

high mortality and morbidity. Therefore, there is a need to develop such materials that efficiently control viral infection. In this context, nanotechnology offers new insights that easily control viral infections. Nanomaterials and biotechnology have exceptional potential that deals with numerous human problems like water treatment, sensors, energy, agriculture, drug delivery, and control of bacteria and viruses (Ashfaq et al., 2017a; Tripathi et al., 2016; Afreen et al., 2018; Ashfaq et al., 2018; Omar et al., 2019a; Chauhan et al., 2020; Sasidharan et al., 2021; Talreja et al., 2021b; Irsad et al., 2020; Chauhan et al., 2021; Afreen et al., 2020; Omar et al., 2019b; Omar et al., 2022; Ashfaq et al., 2021). The applicability of nanomaterials offers a newer platform for the treatment and disinfection of viruses, including COVID-19. Usually, numerous nanomaterials like metal and metal-oxide (Cu, Ag, Zn, and Au) have exceptional antibacterial, antifungal, and antiviral activities, thereby can be extensively used in various biological applications, including nanomedicine. Similarly, metal- and metal-oxide incorporated CNTs, and CNFs, also show themselves to be promising candidates for various biological applications and also increase the biocompatibility compared with the metal- and metal-oxide based nanomaterials (Ashfaq et al., 2016; Singh et al., 2013; Ashfaq et al., 2014; Kumar et al., 2018; Ashfaq et al., 2013, 2017b; Bhadauriya et al., 2018; Mustafa et al., 2011; Ashfaq et al., 2019). There is a continuously increasing concern regarding the control of COVID-19 virus infection. Nanomaterials might target specific parts of the body, and drug molecules distributed throughout the entire body. With the help of nanotechnology, a vaccine can be designed to improve targeted organs or immune cells that enhance the immunological response compared with that of a conventional vaccine. Usually, localized infection is difficult to cure by the conventional vaccine, whereas nanovaccines easily cure it due to the targeted delivery system. On the other hand, nanomaterial-based drug delivery might be improved by the solubility of hydrophobic compounds that improve the stability of therapeutic compounds like proteins and nucleic acid. Moreover, nanomaterials play important roles in the drug delivery system. The nanotechnology-based drug delivery system offers a newer platform to resolve issues associated with conventional drug delivery, thereby increasing interest in controlling viral infections. Furthermore, surface modification might be improved by applicability towards the end application (Muhammad et al., 2020; Serrano-Aroca et al., 2021; Chen and Liang, 2020b; Khoshnevisan et al., 2021; Cardoso et al., 2020; Chang et al., 2021; Almanza-Reyes et al., 2021; Krishnan et al., 2021; Campos et al., 2020; Allawadhi et al., 2021). Numerous studies focus on the synthesis of nanomaterials and their antiviral application, including controlling COVID-19 viruses. For example, Raghuwanshi et al. produced plasmid DNA-loaded chitosan nanoparticles (pDNA-C-NPs). The data suggested that pDNA-C-NPs targeted the bifunctional protein vector and effectively immunized nasal DNA against SARS-CoV infection (Raghuwanshi et al., 2012). Gaikwad et al. synthesized Ag-NPs using fungi and tested antiviral activity against the influenza virus. The data suggested that the Ag-NPs efficiently inhibit the growth of the virus. Moreover, the antiviral activity of the Ag-NPs depends on the different producing systems (Gaikwad et al., 2013). Chen et al. synthesized graphene oxide-incorporated Ag nanoparticles (GO-Ag-NPs) and tested antiviral activity against non-enveloped and enveloped viruses. The data suggested that the prepared GO-Ag-NPs effectively controlled both types of virus infection (Chen et al., 2016). Du et al. synthesized glutathione-capped Ag_2S based nanocluster (Ag_2S-NCs) and tested it against porcine epidemic diarrhoea virus (PEDV). The data suggested that the Ag_2S-NCs effectively control the infection of PEDV within 12h post-infection. **Figure 8.3** shows the plausible mechanism of the Ag_2S-NCs against PEDV as a coronavirus model. The prepared Ag_2S-NCs inhibit the negative sRNA of the virus, regulate the production of the IFN stimulating gene, and express inflammatory cytokines, thereby controlling

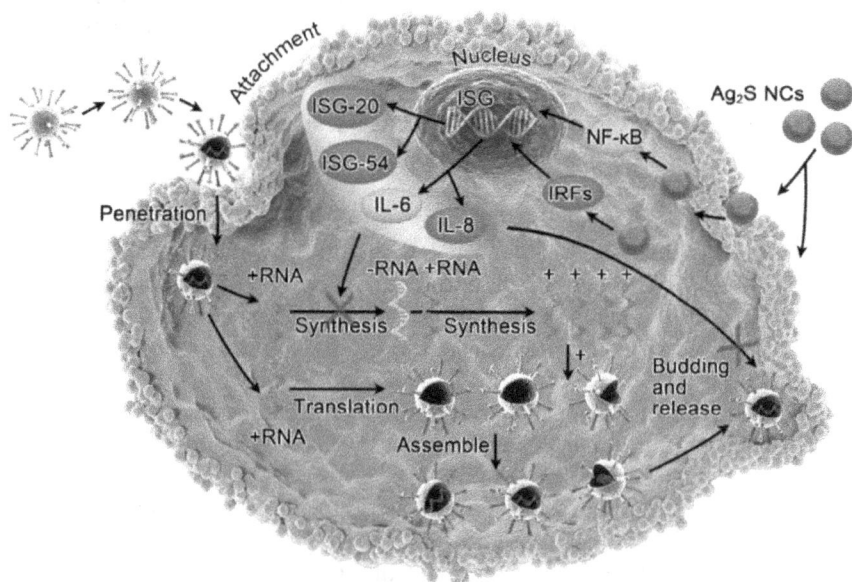

FIGURE 8.3 Plausible antiviral activity of the Ag2S-NCs. The image was taken with permission (Du et al., 2018).

the viral infection (Du et al., 2018). Chang et al. synthesized metal composite (Au, Ag, ZnO, and ClO$_2$-NPs) (TPNT1) and tested it against SARS-CoV infection. The data suggested that the prepared TPNT1-based composite effectively inhibits the viral infection by blocking viral entry (inhibiting viral spike protein to ACE2 inhibitor). Moreover, a prepared TPNT1-based composite reduces the cytopathic effect (Chang et al., 2021). Almanza-Reyes et al. synthesized Ag-NPs and antiviral activity tested against SARS-CoV both in in-vitro and in-vivo tests. The data suggested that the prepared Ag-NPs effectively control the viral infection (Almanza-Reyes et al., 2021). Merkl et al. synthesized Ag-, CuO-, and ZnO-NP-coated filter and tested antiviral activity against SARS-CoV infection. The data suggested that the Ag and CuO-NPs coated filter shows strong antiviral activity, whereas ZnO-NPs coated filter does not show significant antiviral activity (Merkl et al., 2021). Table 8.1 summarized

TABLE 8.1
Different Nanomaterials and Their Antiviral Activity

S.No.	Materials	Virus	Remarks	References
1.	Ag$_2$S-NCs	PEDV	Efficiently suppress the viral activity	(Du et al., 2018)
2.	Viromimetic vaccine	MERS-CoV	Efficiently control the viral infection by neutralization of antibody	(Lin et al., 2019)
3.	AD5-MERS, SP-NP-Al	MERS-CoV	Effectively induce specific immunoglobin G against MERS-CoV infection	(Jung et al., 2018)
4.	CVSP-NP	MERS-CoV, SARS-CoV	Effective neutralization of antibody	(Coleman et al., 2014)
5.	SARS	SARS-CoV	Effective neutralization activity	(Pimentel et al., 2009)
6.	pDNA-C-NPs	SARS-CoV	Effectively immunized nasal DNA	(Raghuwanshi et al., 2012)
7.	GO-Ag-NPs	Enveloped and Non-enveloped virus	Effectively inhibit the growth of virus	(Chen et al., 2016)
8.	Ag-NPs	Influenza Virus	Effectively inhibit the growth of virus	(Gaikwad et al., 2013)
9.	Ag-NPs, CuO-NPs, and ZnO-NPs	SARS-CoV	Strong antiviral effect of Ag, and CuO-NPs. ZnO-NPs does not show any significant antiviral activity	(Merkl et al., 2021)
10.	Metal composite (TPNT1)	SARS-CoV	Efficiently inhibit the viral infection by blocking viral entry	(Chang et al., 2021)
11.	Ag-NPs	SARS-CoV	Prevent viral infection	(Almanza-Reyes et al., 2021)

different nanomaterial-based composites and their antiviral activity especially on the COVID-19 virus. This literature suggested that nanomaterials might be beneficial for controlling the viral infection. Moreover, the incorporation of polymeric composite might increase the therapeutic efficacy. Furthermore, the high biocompatibility of the nanomaterials makes it a promising candidate for controlling viral infections including SARS-CoV.

The exceptional antiviral efficiency of the nanomaterials makes them a suitable candidate for the development of nanovaccines. Numerous studies focus on the nanomaterial-based vaccine for controlling viral infection, especially SARS-CoV. For example, Pimentel et al. produced a prototypic SARS vaccine (Polypeptide nanoparticles with repeated SARS B-epitopes). The data suggested that the produced prototypic SARS vaccine effectively shows neutralization activity (Pimentel et al., 2009). Coleman et al. developed a coronavirus spike protein nanoparticle- (CVSP-NP-) based vaccine for neutralizing mice antibodies. The data suggested that the developed CVSP-NP effectively induced the neutralization of antibodies.

Moreover, these strategies block the entry of the coronavirus and promote antibody targeting (Coleman et al., 2014). Jung et al. developed recombinant-adenovirus-5-MERS-CoV gene (AD5-MERS) and spike protein nanoparticles (NPs) with an aluminium (SP-NP-Al)-based vaccine for controlling viral infection. The data suggested that the developed vaccine induces specific immunoglobin G against MERS-CoV infection. Moreover, immunization with AD5-MERS and boosting with SP-NP-Al might be an effective strategy against MERS-CoV infection (Jung et al., 2018). Lin et al. synthesized a viromimetic vaccine and tested it against the Middle East respiratory syndrome coronavirus (MERS-CoV). The data suggested that the developed nanomaterial-based vaccines effectively control viral infection by neutralizing antibodies and immune responses in mice. Moreover, the developed Viromimetic vaccine shows high biocompatibility that might be a promising tool for controlling viral infection (Lin et al., 2019). These studies suggested that nanomaterial-based vaccines efficiently suppress or inhibit viral infection. Interestingly, high viral efficiency was observed using a nanomaterial-based vaccine compared with that of the conventional vaccine. Therefore, nanomaterial-based vaccines might be a more effective and promising tool to combat pandemic situations (Figure 8.4).

8.5 CONCLUSION

Viral infections are one of the greatest challenges globally that cause a high number of mortality and morbidity. Therefore, there is a need to develop such materials that efficiently control viral infection. The novel strategies, including emerging nanomaterials (NMs) as a drug against the treatment of the virus, can be effective for treating the virus. Moreover, the incorporation of polymeric composite might increase the therapeutic efficacy. Furthermore, the high biocompatibility of the nanomaterials makes them a promising candidate for controlling viral infection, including SARS-CoV. Interestingly, high viral efficiency was observed using nanomaterial-based vaccines compared with that of the conventional vaccine. Therefore, nanomaterial-based vaccines might be a more effective and promising tool to combat pandemic situations.

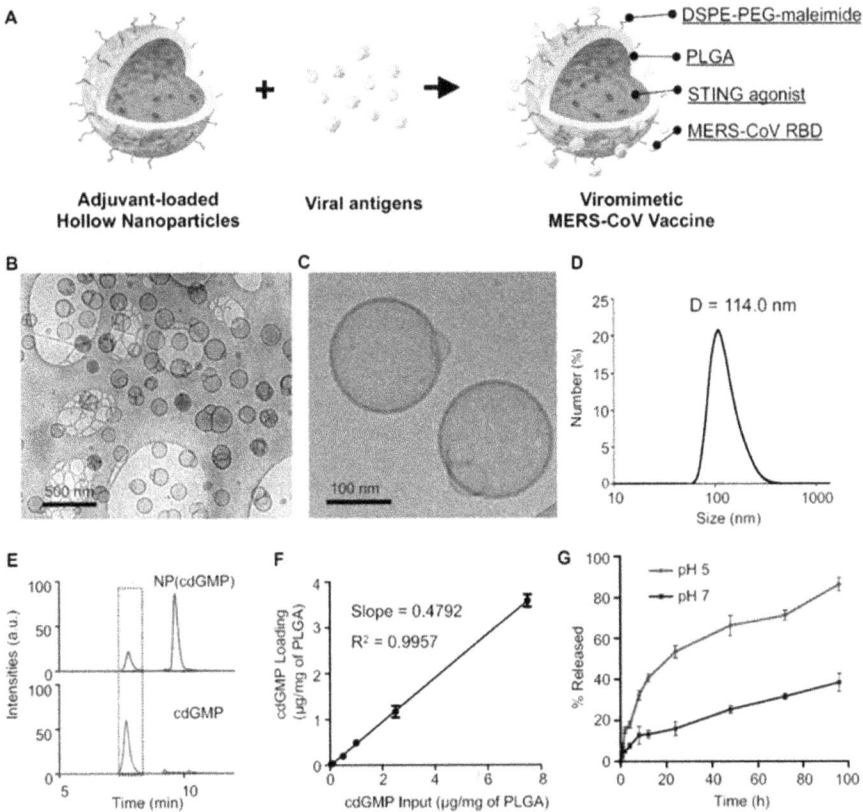

FIGURE 8.4 Schematically representation and characterization of the Viromimetic nano-materials. (A) graphical representation of the Viromimetic nanomaterials based vaccine, (B–C) microscopic images of the nanomaterials, (D) particle size, (E) HPLC, (F) encapsulation efficiency, and (G) in-vitro release behaviour. The image was taken with permission (Lin et al., 2019).

REFERENCES

Abdelrahman, Z., Li, M. & Wang, X. 2020. Comparative review of SARS-CoV-2, SARS-CoV, MERS-CoV, and influenza A respiratory viruses. *Frontiers in Immunology*, 11(2309), 552909.

Afreen, S., Omar, R. A., Talreja, N., Chauhan, D. & Ashfaq, M. 2018. Carbon-based nano-structured materials for energy and environmental remediation applications. *In*: Prasad, R. & Aranda, E. (eds.) *Approaches in Bioremediation: The New Era of Environmental Microbiology and Nanobiotechnology*. Cham: Springer International Publishing, 369–392.

Afreen, S., Talreja, N., Chauhan, D. & Ashfaq, M. 2020. Chapter 15 - Polymer/metal/carbon-based hybrid materials for the detection of heavy metal ions. *In*: Abd-Elsalam, K. A. (ed.) *Multifunctional Hybrid Nanomaterials for Sustainable Agri-Food and Ecosystems*. Elsevier 335–353.

Al-Qahtani, A. A. 2020. Severe acute respiratory syndrome coronavirus 2 (SARS-CoV-2): Emergence, history, basic and clinical aspects. *Saudi Journal of Biological Sciences*, 27(10), pp. 2531–2538.

Alberti, S. & Jágerská, J. 2021. Sol-gel thin film processing for integrated waveguide sensors. *Frontiers in Materials*, 8(23), 629822.

Allawadhi, P., Singh, V., Khurana, A., Khurana, I., Allwadhi, S., Kumar, P., Banothu, A. K., Thalugula, S., Barani, P. J., Naik, R. R. & Bharani, K. K. 2021. Silver nanoparticle-based multifunctional approach for combating COVID-19. *Sensors International*, 2, p. 100101.

Almanza-Reyes, H., Moreno, S., Plascencia-López, I., Alvarado-Vera, M., Patrón-Romero, L., Borrego, B., Reyes-Escamilla, A., Valencia-Manzo, D., Brun, A., Pestryakov, A. & Bogdanchikova, N. 2021. Evaluation of silver nanoparticles for the prevention of SARS-CoV-2 infection in health workers: In vitro and in vivo. *PLOS ONE*, 16(8), p. e0256401.

Amighian, J., Mozaffari, M. & Nasr, B. 2006. Preparation of nano-sized manganese ferrite ($MnFe_2O_4$) via coprecipitation method. *Physica Status Solidi (C)*, 3(9), pp. 3188–3192.

Ani, M. H., Kamarudin, M. A., Ramlan, A. H., Ismail, E., Sirat, M. S., Mohamed, M. A. & Azam, M. A. 2018. A critical review on the contributions of chemical and physical factors toward the nucleation and growth of large-area graphene. *Journal of Materials Science*, 53(10), pp. 7095–7111.

Ashfaq, M., Khan, S. & Verma, N. 2014. Synthesis of PVA-CAP-based biomaterial in situ dispersed with Cu nanoparticles and carbon micro-nanofibers for antibiotic drug delivery applications. *Biochemical Engineering Journal*, 90, pp. 79–89.

Ashfaq, M., Singh, S., Sharma, A. & Verma, N. 2013. Cytotoxic evaluation of the hierarchical web of carbon micronanofibers. *Industrial and Engineering Chemistry Research*, 52(12), pp. 4672–4682.

Ashfaq, M., Talreja, N., Chauhan, D., Rodríguez, C. A., Mera, A. C. & Mangalaraja, R. V. 2021. A novel bimetallic (Fe/Bi)-povidone-iodine micro-flowers composite for photocatalytic and antibacterial applications. *Journal of Photochemistry and Photobiology B: Biology*, 219, p. 112204.

Ashfaq, M., Talreja, N., Chuahan, D. & Srituravanich, W. 2019. Carbon nanostructure-based materials: A novel tool for detection of Alzheimer's disease. *In*: Ashraf, G. M. & Alexiou, A. (eds.) *Biological, Diagnostic and Therapeutic Advances in Alzheimer's Disease: Non-pharmacological Therapies for Alzheimer's Disease*. Singapore: Springer Singapore, 71–89.

Ashfaq, M., Verma, N. & Khan, S. 2016. Copper/zinc bimetal nanoparticles-dispersed carbon nanofibers: A novel potential antibiotic material. *Materials Science and Engineering: C*, 59, pp. 938–947.

Ashfaq, M., Verma, N. & Khan, S. 2017a. Carbon nanofibers as a micronutrient carrier in plants: Efficient translocation and controlled release of Cu nanoparticles. *Environmental Science: Nano*, 4(1), pp. 138–148.

Ashfaq, M., Verma, N. & Khan, S. 2017b. Highly effective Cu/Zn-carbon micro/nanofiber-polymer nanocomposite-based wound dressing biomaterial against the P. aeruginosa multi- and extensively drug-resistant strains. *Materials Science and Engineering: C*, 77, pp. 630–641.

Ashfaq, M., Verma, N. & Khan, S. 2018. Novel polymeric composite grafted with metal nanoparticle-dispersed CNFs as a chemiresistive non-destructive fruit sensor material. *Materials Chemistry and Physics*, 217, pp. 216–227.

Bhadauriya, P., Mamtani, H., Ashfaq, M., Raghav, A., Teotia, A. K., Kumar, A. & Verma, N. 2018. Synthesis of yeast-immobilized and copper nanoparticle-dispersed carbon nanofiber-based diabetic wound dressing material: Simultaneous control of glucose and bacterial infections. *ACS Applied Bio Materials*, 1(2), pp. 246–258.

Cai, Z., Liu, B., Zou, X. & Cheng, H.-M. 2018. Chemical vapor deposition growth and applications of two-dimensional materials and their heterostructures. *Chemical Reviews*, 118(13), pp. 6091–6133.

Campos, E. V. R., Pereira, A. E. S., de Oliveira, J. L., Carvalho, L. B., Guilger-Casagrande, M., de Lima, R. & Fraceto, L. F. 2020. How can nanotechnology help to combat COVID-19? Opportunities and urgent need. *Journal of Nanobiotechnology*, 18(1), p. 125.

Cardoso, V. M. D. O., Moreira, B. J., Comparetti, E. J., Sampaio, I., Ferreira, L. M. B., Lins, P. M. P. & Zucolotto, V. 2020. Is nanotechnology helping in the fight against COVID-19? *Frontiers in Nanotechnology*, 2, p. 4.

Carvalho, A. P. A. & Conte-Junior, C. A. 2021. Recent advances on nanomaterials to COVID-19 management: A systematic review on antiviral/virucidal agents and mechanisms of SARS-CoV-2 inhibition/inactivation. *Global Challenges*, 5(5), p. 2000115.

Chang, S.-Y., Huang, K.-Y., Chao, T.-L., Kao, H.-C., Pang, Y.-H., Lu, L., Chiu, C.-L., Huang, H.-C., Cheng, T.-J. R., Fang, J.-M. & Yang, P.-C. 2021. Nanoparticle composite TPNT1 is effective against SARS-CoV-2 and influenza viruses. *Scientific Reports*, 11(1), p. 8692.

Chauhan, D., Afreen, S., Talreja, N. & Ashfaq, M. 2020. Chapter 8 - Multifunctional copper polymer-based nanocomposite for environmental and agricultural applications. *In*: Abd-Elsalam, K. A. (ed.) *Multifunctional Hybrid Nanomaterials for Sustainable Agri-Food and Ecosystems*. Elsevier 189–211.

Chauhan, D., Ashfaq, M., Talreja, N. & Managalraja, R. V. 2021. 2D materials for environment, energy, and biomedical applications. *Journal of Biomedical Research & Environmental Sciences*, 2(10), pp. 977–984.

Chauhan, D., Talreja, N. & Ashfaq, M. 2021. Chapter 13 - Nanoadsorbents for wastewater remediation. *In*: Abd-Elsalam, K. A. & Zahid, M. (eds.) *Aquananotechnology*. Elsevier 273–290.

Chauhan, Divya, Talreja, Neetu, Ashfaq, Mohammad, Mera, Adriana C & Rodríguez, Carlos A, 2021 *Polymeric Nanocomposite for Nanoremediation: Laboratory to Land Approach, Pesticide Contamination in Freshwater and Soil Environs*. Apple Academic Press, 343–359.

Chen, L. & Liang, J. 2020a. An overview of functional nanoparticles as novel emerging antiviral therapeutic agents. *Materials Science and Engineering: Part C*, 112, p. 110924.

Chen, L. & Liang, J. 2020b. An overview of functional nanoparticles as novel emerging antiviral therapeutic agents. *Materials Science and Engineering: C, Materials for Biological Applications*, 112, pp. 110924–110924.

Chen, Y.-N., Hsueh, Y.-H., Hsieh, C.-T., Tzou, D.-Y. & Chang, P.-L. 2016. Antiviral activity of graphene-silver nanocomposites against non-enveloped and enveloped viruses. *International Journal of Environmental Research and Public Health*, 13(4), pp. 430–430.

Coleman, C. M., Liu, Y. V., Mu, H., Taylor, J. K., Massare, M., Flyer, D. C., Smith, G. E. & Frieman, M. B. 2014. Purified coronavirus spike protein nanoparticles induce coronavirus neutralizing antibodies in mice. *Vaccine*, 32(26), pp. 3169–3174.

Danks, A. E., Hall, S. R. & Schnepp, Z. 2016. The evolution of 'sol–gel' chemistry as a technique for materials synthesis. *Materials Horizons*, 3(2), pp. 91–112.

Ding, Y., Jiang, Y., Xu, F., Yin, J., Ren, H., Zhuo, Q., Long, Z. & Zhang, P. 2010. Preparation of nano-structured LiFePO$_4$/graphene composites by co-precipitation method. *Electrochemistry Communications*, 12(1), pp. 10–13.

Du, T., Liang, J., Dong, N., Lu, J., Fu, Y., Fang, L., Xiao, S. & Han, H. 2018. Glutathione-capped Ag$_2$S nanoclusters inhibit coronavirus proliferation through blockage of viral RNA synthesis and budding. *ACS Applied Materials and Interfaces*, 10(5), pp. 4369–4378.

Gaikwad, S., Ingle, A., Gade, A., Rai, M., Falanga, A., Incoronato, N., Russo, L., Galdiero, S. & Galdiero, M. 2013. Antiviral activity of mycosynthesized silver nanoparticles against herpes simplex virus and human parainfluenza virus type 3. *International Journal of Nanomedicine*, 8, pp. 4303–4314.

Galdiero, S., Falanga, A., Vitiello, M., Cantisani, M., Marra, V. & Galdiero, M. 2011. Silver nanoparticles as potential antiviral agents. *Molecules*, 16(10), 8894–918.

Hench, L. L. & West, J. K. 1990. The sol-gel process. *Chemical Reviews*, 90(1), pp. 33–72.

Ibrahim Fouad, G. 2021. A proposed insight into the anti-viral potential of metallic nanoparticles against novel coronavirus disease-19 (COVID-19). *Bulletin of the National Research Centre*, 45(1), p. 36.

Irsad, Talreja, N., Chauhan, D., Rodríguez, C. A., Mera, A. C. & Ashfaq, M. 2020. Nanocarriers: An emerging tool for micronutrient delivery in plants. *In*: Aftab, T. & Hakeem, K. R. (eds.) *Plant Micronutrients: Deficiency and Toxicity Management*. Cham: Springer International Publishing, 373–387.

Jayaweera, M., Perera, H., Gunawardana, B. & Manatunge, J. 2020. Transmission of COVID-19 virus by droplets and aerosols: A critical review on the unresolved dichotomy. *Environmental Research*, 188, pp. 109819–109819.

Jones, K. E., Patel, N. G., Levy, M. A., Storeygard, A., Balk, D., Gittleman, J. L. & Daszak, P. 2008. Global trends in emerging infectious diseases. *Nature*, 451(7181), pp. 990–993.

Jung, S.-Y., Kang, K. W., Lee, E.-Y., Seo, D.-W., Kim, H.-L., Kim, H., Kwon, T., Park, H.-L., Kim, H., Lee, S.-M. & Nam, J.-H. 2018. Heterologous prime–boost vaccination with adenoviral vector and protein nanoparticles induces both Th1 and Th2 responses against Middle East respiratory syndrome coronavirus. *Vaccine*, 36(24), pp. 3468–3476.

Kevadiya, B. D., Machhi, J., Herskovitz, J., Oleynikov, M. D., Blomberg, W. R., Bajwa, N., Soni, D., Das, S., Hasan, M., Patel, M., Senan, A. M., Gorantla, S., McMillan, J., Edagwa, B., Eisenberg, R., Gurumurthy, C. B., Reid, S. P. M., Punyadeera, C., Chang, L. & Gendelman, H. E. 2021. Diagnostics for SARS-CoV-2 infections. *Nature Materials*, 20(5), pp. 593–605.

Khoshnevisan, K., Maleki, H. & Baharifar, H. 2021. Nanobiocide based-silver nanomaterials upon coronaviruses: Approaches for preventing viral infections. *Nanoscale Research Letters*, 16(1), p. 100.

Klompas, M., Baker, M. A. & Rhee, C. 2020. Airborne transmission of SARS-CoV-2: Theoretical considerations and available evidence. *JAMA*, 324(5), pp. 441–442.

Kragstrup, T. W., Singh, H. S., Grundberg, I., Nielsen, A. L.-L., Rivellese, F., Mehta, A., Goldberg, M. B., Filbin, M. R., Qvist, P. & Bibby, B. M. 2021. Plasma ACE2 predicts outcome of COVID-19 in hospitalized patients. *PLOS ONE*, 16(6), p. e0252799.

Krishnan, S., Thirunavukarasu, A., Jha, N. K., Gahtori, R., Roy, A. S., Dholpuria, S., Kesari, K. K., Singh, S. K., Dua, K. & Gupta, P. K. 2021. Nanotechnology-based therapeutic formulations in the battle against animal coronaviruses: An update. *Journal of Nanoparticle Research*, 23(10), p. 229.

Kumar, R., Ashfaq, M. & Verma, N. 2018. Synthesis of novel PVA–starch formulation-supported Cu–Zn nanoparticle carrying carbon nanofibers as a nanofertilizer: Controlled release of micronutrients. *Journal of Materials Science*, 53(10), pp. 7150–7164.

Kumar, R., Nayak, M., Sahoo, G. C., Pandey, K., Sarkar, M. C., Ansari, Y., Das, V. N. R., Topno, R. K., Bhawna, Madhukar, M. & Das, P. 2019. Iron oxide nanoparticles based antiviral activity of H1N1 influenza A virus. *Journal of Infection and Chemotherapy*, 25(5), pp. 325–329.

LaGrow, A. P., Besenhard, M. O., Hodzic, A., Sergides, A., Bogart, L. K., Gavriilidis, A. & Thanh, N. T. K. 2019. Unravelling the growth mechanism of the co-precipitation of iron oxide nanoparticles with the aid of synchrotron X-ray diffraction in solution. *Nanoscale*, 11(14), pp. 6620–6628.

Leung, N. H. L. 2021. Transmissibility and transmission of respiratory viruses. *Nature Reviews in Microbiology*, 19(8), pp. 528–545.

Lin, L. C., Huang, C. Y., Yao, B. Y., Lin, J. C., Agrawal, A., Algaissi, A., Peng, B. H., Liu, Y. H., Huang, P. H., Juang, R. H., Chang, Y. C., Tseng, C. T., Chen, H. W. & Hu, C. J. 2019. Viromimetic STING agonist-loaded hollow polymeric nanoparticles for safe and effective vaccination against Middle East respiratory syndrome coronavirus, 29(28), p. 1807616.

Livage, J. 1997. Sol-gel processes. *Current Opinion in Solid State and Materials Science*, 2(2), pp. 132–138.

Mehranfar, A. & Izadyar, M. 2020. Theoretical design of functionalized gold nanoparticles as antiviral agents against severe acute respiratory syndrome coronavirus 2 (SARS-CoV-2). *The Journal of Physical Chemistry Letters*, 11(24), pp. 10284–10289.

Merkl, P., Long, S., McInerney, G. M. & Sotiriou, G. A. 2021. Antiviral activity of silver, copper oxide and zinc oxide nanoparticle coatings against SARS-CoV-2. *Nanomaterials*, 11(5), 1312.

Muhammad, W., Zhai, Z. & Gao, C. 2020. Antiviral activity of nanomaterials against coronaviruses. *Macromolecular Bioscience*, 20(10), p. 2000196.

Muñoz, R. & Gómez-Aleixandre, C. 2013. Review of CVD synthesis of graphene. *Chemical Vapor Deposition*, 19(10-11-12), pp. 297–322.

Mustafa, S., Khan, H. M., Shukla, I., Shujatullah, F., Shahid, M., Ashfaq, M. & Azam, A. 2011. Effect of ZnO nanoparticles on ESBL producing Escherichia coli & Klebsiella spp. *Eastern Journal of Medicine*, 16(4), pp. 253–257.

Nickels, L. 2020. Antiviral boost for nanoparticles. *Metal Powder Report*, 75(6), pp. 330–333.

Omar, R. A., Afreen, S., Talreja, N., Chauhan, D. & Ashfaq, M. 2019a. Impact of nanomaterials in plant systems. *In*: Prasad, R. (ed.) *Plant Nanobionics: Volume 1, Advances in the Understanding of Nanomaterials Research and Applications*. Cham: Springer International Publishing, 117–140.

Omar, R. A., Afreen, S., Talreja, N., Chauhan, D., Ashfaq, M. & Srituravanich, W. 2019b. Impact of nanomaterials on the microbial system. *In*: Prasad, R. (ed.) *Microbial Nanobionics: Volume 1, State-of-the-Art*. Cham: Springer International Publishing, 141–158.

Omar, R. A., Chauhan, D., Talreja, N., Mangalaraja, R. V. & Ashfaq, M. 2022. Chapter 12 - Vegetables waste for biosynthesis of various nanoparticles. *In*: Abd-Elsalam, K. A., Periakaruppan, R. & Rajeshkumar, S. (eds.) *Agri-Waste and Microbes for Production of Sustainable Nanomaterials*. Elsevier, 281–298.

Parashar, M., Shukla, V. K. & Singh, R. 2020. Metal oxides nanoparticles via sol–gel method: A review on synthesis, characterization and applications. *Journal of Materials Science: Materials in Electronics*, 31(5), pp. 3729–3749.

Park, S. E. 2020. Epidemiology, virology, and clinical features of severe acute respiratory syndrome -coronavirus-2 (SARS-CoV-2; coronavirus disease-19). *Clin Exp Pediatr*, 63(4), pp. 119–124.

Peplow, M. 2021. Nanotechnology offers alternative ways to fight COVID-19 pandemic with antivirals. *Nature Biotechnology*, 39(10), pp. 1172–1174.

Pimentel, T. A., Yan, Z., Jeffers, S. A., Holmes, K. V., Hodges, R. S. & Burkhard, P. 2009. Peptide nanoparticles as novel immunogens: Design and analysis of a prototypic severe acute respiratory syndrome vaccine. *Chemical Biology and Drug Design*, 73(1), pp. 53–61.

Proal, A. D. & Van Elzakker, M. B. 2021. Long COVID or post-acute sequelae of COVID-19 (PASC): An overview of biological factors that may contribute to persistent symptoms. *Frontiers in Microbiology*, 12(1494).

Raghuwanshi, D., Mishra, V., Das, D., Kaur, K. & Suresh, M. R. 2012. Dendritic cell targeted chitosan nanoparticles for nasal DNA immunization against SARS CoV nucleocapsid protein. *Molecular Pharmaceutics*, 9(4), pp. 946–956.

Rohr, J. R., Barrett, C. B., Civitello, D. J., Craft, M. E., Delius, B., DeLeo, G. A., Hudson, P. J., Jouanard, N., Nguyen, K. H., Ostfeld, R. S., Remais, J. V., Riveau, G., Sokolow, S. H. & Tilman, D. 2019. Emerging human infectious diseases and the links to global food production. *Nature Sustainability*, 2(6), pp. 445–456.

Sasidharan, V., Sachan, D., Chauhan, D., Talreja, N. & Ashfaq, M. 2021. Three-dimensional (3D) polymer—Metal–carbon framework for efficient removal of chemical and biological contaminants. *Scientific Reports*, 11(1), p. 7708.

Schwander, M. & Partes, K. 2011. A review of diamond synthesis by CVD processes. *Diamond and Related Materials*, 20(9), pp. 1287–1301.

Serrano-Aroca, Á., Takayama, K., Tuñón-Molina, A., Seyran, M., Hassan, S. S., Pal Choudhury, P., Uversky, V. N., Lundstrom, K., Adadi, P., Palù, G., Aljabali, A. A. A., Chauhan, G., Kandimalla, R., Tambuwala, M. M., Lal, A., Abd El-Aziz, T. M., Sherchan, S., Barh, D., Redwan, E. M., Bazan, N. G., Mishra, Y. K., Uhal, B. D. & Brufsky, A. 2021. Carbon-based nanomaterials: Promising antiviral agents to combat COVID-19 in the microbial-resistant era. *ACS Nano*, 15(5), pp. 8069–8086.

Sharma, A., Tiwari, S., Deb, M. K. & Marty, J. L. 2020. Severe acute respiratory syndrome coronavirus-2 (SARS-CoV-2): A global pandemic and treatment strategies. *International Journal of Antimicrobial Agents*, 56(2), pp. 106054–106054.

Shionoiri, N., Sato, T., Fujimori, Y., Nakayama, T., Nemoto, M., Matsunaga, T. & Tanaka, T. 2012. Investigation of the antiviral properties of copper iodide nanoparticles against feline calicivirus. *Journal of Bioscience and Bioengineering*, 113(5), pp. 580–586.

Singh, S., Ashfaq, M., Singh, R. K., Joshi, H. C., Srivastava, A., Sharma, A. & Verma, N. 2013. Preparation of surfactant-mediated silver and copper nanoparticles dispersed in hierarchical carbon micro-nanofibers for antibacterial applications. *New Biotechnology*, 30(6), pp. 656–665.

Sultana, A., Talreja, N., Chauhan, D. & Ashfaq, M. 2021. Chapter 4 – Nanotechnology-based biofortification: A plant–soil interaction modulator/enhancer. *In*: Aftab, T. & Hakeem, K. R. (eds.) *Frontiers in Plant-Soil Interaction*. Academic Press, pp. 83–105.

Talreja, N., Afreen, S., Ashfaq, M., Chauhan, D., Mera, A. C., Rodríguez, C. A. & Mangalaraja, R. V. 2021a. Bimetal (Fe/Zn) doped BiOI photocatalyst: An effective photodegradation of tetracycline and bacteria. *Chemosphere*, 280, p. 130803.

Talreja, N., Ashfaq, M., Chauhan, D., Mera, A. C. & Rodríguez, C. A. 2021b. Strategic doping approach of the Fe–BiOI microstructure: An improved photodegradation efficiency of tetracycline. *ACS Omega*, 6(2), pp. 1575–1583.

Talreja, N., Ashfaq, M., Chauhan, D., Mera, A. C., Rodríguez, C. A. & Mangalaraja, R. V. 2021c. A Zn-doped BiOI microsponge-based photocatalyst material for complete photodegradation of environmental contaminants. *New Journal of Chemistry*, 45(39), pp. 18412–18420.

Tang, D., Comish, P. & Kang, R. 2020. The hallmarks of COVID-19 disease. *PLOS Pathogens*, 16(5), p. e1008536.

Trefry, J. C. & Wooley, D. P. 2012. Rapid assessment of antiviral activity and cytotoxicity of silver nanoparticles using a novel application of the tetrazolium-based colorimetric assay. *Journal of Virological Methods*, 183(1), pp. 19–24.

Tripathi, K. M., Tyagi, A., Ashfaq, M. & Gupta, R. K. 2016. Temperature dependent, shape variant synthesis of photoluminescent and biocompatible carbon nanostructures from almond husk for applications in dye removal. *RSC Advances*, 6(35), pp. 29545–29553.

V'kovski, P., Kratzel, A., Steiner, S., Stalder, H. & Thiel, V. 2021. Coronavirus biology and replication: Implications for SARS-CoV-2. *Nature Reviews in Microbiology*, 19(3), pp. 155–170.

Vodnar, D. C., Mitrea, L., Călinoiu, L. F., Szabo, K. & Ştefănescu, B. E. 2020. Removal of bacteria, viruses, and other microbial entities by means of nanoparticles. *In*: Baia, L., Pap, Z., Hernadi, K. & Baia, M. (eds.) *Advanced Nanostructures for Environmental Health*. Elsevier, 465–491.

Index

For Product Safety Concerns and Information please contact our EU
representative GPSR@taylorandfrancis.com
Taylor & Francis Verlag GmbH, Kaufingerstraße 24, 80331 München, Germany

www.ingramcontent.com/pod-product-compliance
Lightning Source LLC
Chambersburg PA
CBHW070725220326
41598CB00024BA/3298